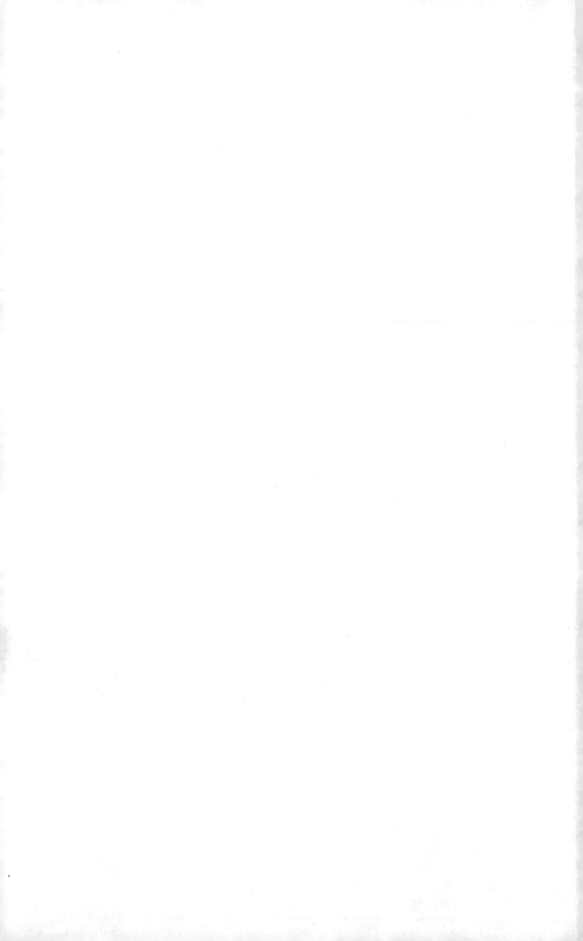

Advances in Clinical Neuropsychology

Volume 1

Advances in Clinical Neuropsychology

Volume 1

Edited by
Gerald Goldstein

Veterans Administration Medical Center and
University of Pittsburgh School of Medicine
Pittsburgh, Pennsylvania

Plenum Press • New York and London

ISBN 0-306-41502-X

ACKNOWLEDGMENTS

The editor would like to acknowledge the support of the Department of Psychiatry of the University of Pittsburgh and the Western Psychiatric Institute and Clinic for sponsoring the conference which stimulated the development of this volume.

The following individuals acknowledge the support of the Veterans Administration for the research described in their work: Nancy Helm-Estabrooks, Gerald Goldstein, François Boller, Youngjai Kim, and Nelson Butters and his collaborators. Dr. Butters and his collaborators also wish to acknowledge support of their work by a grant from NIAAA (#00187). Edward M. Stricker and Michael J. Zigmond wish to acknowledge that their work was supported, in part, by USPHS grants MH-20620, MH-29670, MH-00058, MH-00338, MH-30915, and NSMH-16359. Some of this work was carried out in collaboration with A. Acheson, P. Cooper, M. Friedman, T. Heffner, L. Kennedy, D. Levitan, C. Saller, A. Snyder, A. Swerdloff, and J. Van Zoeren. Technical assistance for Drs. Stricker and Zigmond was provided by L. Howdyshell, D. McKeag, S. Wuerthele, and J. Yen.

CONTENTS

INTRODUCTION

Gerald Goldstein

Highland Drive Veterans Administration
Medical Center
Pittsburgh, PA

This first, of hopefully many, volumes reporting on the progress
of clinical neuropsychology as a science and profession, provides an
overview of the field through a presentation of selected topics which
are presently felt to be of major importance to the discipline. A
few of the chapters are primarily concerned with clinical and professional matters, while others are more basic science oriented. In the
first chapter, Oscar Parsons provides us with a comprehensive review
of recent developments in the field, covering both clinical and experimental matters. It is clear from this chapter that neuropsychology has proliferated greatly in the past several years, and has
become both a specialty of clinical practice, as well as a separately
identifiable scientific subdiscipline. The book was edited with the
idea that it should sample from both the basic science and clinical
application aspects of the field. Thus, we have Dr. Stricker and
Dr. Zigmond's chapter on animal models of recovery of brain function,
and the chapter by Dr. Butters and his colleagues reporting on recent
laboratory findings concerning memory abilities in amnesic patients.
The review by Dr. Boller and his colleagues provides a consideration
of both the experimental and the clinical literature pertinent to
Alzheimer disease and related dementias, while the chapters by Dr.
Helm-Estabrooks and Dr. Holland, and myself, cover topics associated
with clinical assessment and treatment.

    In the following pages of this introductory material, we will
try to provide the reader who may be unfamiliar with the discipline
some general description of its major emphases and areas of concern.
We would hope that this material may be considered as prefatory to
this volume, and perhaps the series as a whole, which will go on to
consider topics of more specialized areas of interest. Such matters
as a definition of the profession, its history, and its major content

areas will be considered here, but only in an attempt to provide an
overall orientation to the field.

Clinical Neuropsychology and Clinical Neuropsychologists

While the word "psychology" is included in the term "clinical
neuropsychology," the field is actually an interdisciplinary one.
The International Neuropsychological Society, one of the major organizations in the field, has many members who are not psychologists,
but who may be physicians, educators, speech pathologists, rehabilitation specialists, and so on. There are many active clinical neuropsychologists who are trained as neurologists. Others are psychiatrists or speech pathologists. Within psychology, many clinical neuropsychologists are not clinical psychologists, but may be trained
in such areas as physiological, developmental, or experimental psychology. The focuses of interest are relations between the human
brain and behavior, and on the behavioral pathology which stems from
the great variety of neurological disorders. There is a group of
psychologists who are professionally identified as practicing clinical neuropsychologists, but the field as a whole, as well as the
orientation of this series, may be viewed in terms of clinical neuropsychology as an interdisciplinary endeavor.

The clinical focus of the field has traditionally been on the
brain damaged patient who is assessed and treated on the basis of
current knowledge in the area of human brain-behavior relationships.
Some neuropsychologists have turned their interests toward psychiatric patients, and some toward studies of normal individuals, but
the theme of brain-behavior relationships is always at the core of
the clinical or scientific work done. Thus, neuropsychologists may
find themselves in general medical or psychiatric hospitals, rehabilitation centers, educational settings, or university laboratories.
They may function on multidisciplinary teams with neurologists, neurosurgeons, teachers, rehabilitation specialists, or laboratory scientists, depending on the setting in which they find themselves.

While clinical neuropsychologists are probably best known for
the specialized tests they use to examine brain damaged patients,
many members of the discipline are heavily involved with treatment
and rehabilitation. Others function essentially as basic scientists
or clinical researchers. Within the realm of assessment, there is
a variety of tests and testing philosophies and approaches (Lezak,
1983), and an important interface with other methods of diagnosing
brain disorders. Some commentators have taken the view that the
assessment component of clinical neuropsychology is becoming obso-
lescent with the advent of the new brain imaging techniques, the
first of which was the CT Scan. While this view is at odds with
the expanding nature of the field, as described in this volume by
Dr. Parsons, there nevertheless needs to be some understanding of

the nature of the interface, and of the role of neuropsychological assessment <u>vis</u> <u>a</u> <u>vis</u> the other diagnostic methods.

While most neuropsychologists are concerned with some aspect of diagnosis, it can be said that their diagnostic work is done by examining what the brain does, rather than by examining the brain directly. That is, diagnosis is achieved largely through an analysis of function, rather than through, for example, the imaging of brain structures. While such techniques as the electroencephalogram (EEG) also look at function, neuropsychologists generally define function in terms of behavior, rather than physiological aspects of brain activity. Thus, function in terms of operating on the environment is really the focus of interest. The realm of behavior which interests most neuropsychologists generally has to do with cognitive processes and perceptual and motor skills. The area of cognitive processes is typically divided into general intellectual functioning, memory, language, nonverbal abilities such as visual-spatial skills, and conceptual abilities. The perceptual processes examined tend to be higher level visual, auditory and tactile skills. Thus, for example, the neuropsychologist would be more interested in the integration of visual impressions into meaningful percepts than in vision or visual acuity <u>per se</u>. Motor skills range from the ability to perform simple movements of the limbs, to complex constructional activity and the use of movement in communication and other cognitive processes. Impairments of these behaviors are often associated with some form of brain dysfunction, which may be localized or generalized in nature and that may reflect the consequences of a variety of brain disorders. Thus, the brain damaged patient may reflect his/her neurological deficit in the form of general loss of intellectual function or in the loss of the ability to use some modality such as the capacity to organize visual impressions or speech, or as a combination of intellectual and modality impairment. As Teuber (1959) has perhaps most forcefully pointed out, the deficits are often quite subtle and specific, and cannot be detected through casual contact or examination. It is felt that some form of detailed neuropsychological examination provides the most effective way of eliciting the individual patient's pattern of preserved and impaired abilities.

Deficits in the areas outlined above are often patterned in nature and may form syndromes, or sets of symptoms which characteristically occur together. Within each of the functional areas mentioned above, there is a number of syndromes that are seen in patients with the appropriate type of brain disorder. Perhaps this point can be best illustrated with an example. If the impairment is in the language area, the general deficit is known as aphasia. Within aphasia, however, there are numerous subtypes such as "Broca's Aphasia" or "Conduction Aphasia." Each of these types constitute an aphasic syndrome and may be identified through the pattern of the patient's impaired and preserved language abilities. The distinction among these subtypes are of clinical significance in that

they relate to selecting the most appropriate form of treatment, as
well as to the localization of the brain lesion which produced the
aphasia. In assessing an aphasic patient, one important task of the
neuropsychologist is that of identifying the aphasic syndrome the
patient exhibits. Many specialized tests are available for this purpose (Goodglass & Kaplan, 1972; Kertesz, 1979), and are known as
aphasia batteries or examinations. Administration of these tests
may reveal, for example, that the patient has a halting, labored,
impoverished speech and difficulty reading, but understands spoken
language quite well; or alternatively, that the patient's speech is
fluent and smooth, but he has no comprehension of what is being said.
These different forms of aphasia generally stem from lesions in different areas of the brain, and clearly cannot be treated in the same
manner.

In addition to language, neuropsychologists typically look at
syndromes in the following areas: (1) memory; (2) visuoperceptive,
visuospatial and visuoconstructive disorders; (3) body schema disturbances; (4) apraxia or impairment of purposive movement; and,
(5) dementia or impairment of intellectual ability. Thus, future
volumes of this series may be devoted to memory or to disorders of
movement, since each of these areas, as well as the others mentioned,
represent specialized interests within clinical neuropsychology, each
having its own research literature and clinical folklore. Indeed,
some clinical neuropsychologists have international reputations as
specialists in one or more of these areas. From a somewhat different
perspective, neuropsychologists may focus their interests along
specific disorders, rather than syndrome lines. Thus, some neuropsychologists have particular interests and expertise in such disorders as alcoholism or multiple sclerosis or Alzheimer disease.
The literature abounds with papers, chapters and books on such topics
as the neuropsychology of alcoholism (Butters & Cermak, 1980;
Goldstein & Neuringer, 1976), or neuropsychological aspects of multiple sclerosis (Ross & Reitan, 1955; Goldstein & Shelly, 1977).

There appears to be a growing interest in neuropsychology with
regard to groups other than brain damaged patients. There is a great
deal of interest in patients with functional psychiatric disorders
(e.g., Gruzelier & Flor-Henry, 1979) and in the applications of neuropsychology to functioning within the normal range (Kimura & Durnford, 1974). The interest in psychiatric patients is based on the
belief that several of the major psychiatric disorders may be associated in some way with impaired brain function. Indeed, a book has
recently appeared entitled "Schizophrenia as a Brain Disease" (Henn
& Nasrallah, 1982), thereby reflecting the growing interest in the
biological aspects of the functional psychiatric disorders. Interests in this area reflect both an attempt to gain some theoretical
understanding of brain function in these disorders and to find some
means of distinguishing between the cognitive functioning of psychiatric patients, as opposed to patients with structural brain damage

(Heaton & Crowley, 1981). The small, but growing, interest in the clinical neuropsychology of normal individuals relates to such matters as using various models of brain function to evaluate intellectual and learning ability and the use of neuropsychological tests in vocational and educational planning.

Clinical neuropsychology plays two major roles in the area of treatment. First, neuropsychological tests are often used to evaluate the efficacy of some form of treatment. Recently, there has been a major interest in the pharmacological treatment of dementia with a series of compounds thought to be effective in enhancing memory and learning abilities (Reisberg, Ferris & Gershon, 1980; Ferris et al., 1982). Many tests of memory and other cognitive abilities have frequently been used within the framework of various drug research designs to evaluate change in performance level. Some neuropsychologists, however, have become directly involved in treatment (Goldstein & Ruthven, 1983), and have formulated and assessed behavioral treatments based on neuropsychological principles. Thus, in addition to the area in which such treatment was a traditional modality, aphasia and other speech and language disorders, there is now an increasing interest in memory training and training in other cognitive skills. Dr. Parsons reviews this work in his chapter.

A Brief History

Some scholars would mark the beginning of clinical neuropsychology with Paul Broca's report made during the 1860's, of a patient who lost the ability to speak following damage to the anterior portion of his left cerebral hemisphere (Broca, 1861). The relationship found between the anterior portion of the left hemisphere and expressive speech may be viewed as the first discovered principle of clinical neuropsychology. This beginning led to a large number of studies, accomplished originally in Europe and later in the United States, relating areas of localized brain damage to discrete behavioral functions. This movement, now generally known as behavioral neurology, was extremely important for clinical neuropsychology during its formative years, but later became intertwined with the psychometrics and clinical psychology which developed mainly in the United States. Specifically, clinical psychologists became interested in assessing brain damaged patients, particularly those in psychiatric facilities, as part of their general assessment practices. Before the development of what are now known as neuropsychological tests, all they could resort to were the generally available psychometric instruments, notably standardized tests of intelligence and projective tests, such as the Rorschach technique. Thus, while the behavioral neurologists tended to rely largely on extensions of the neurological examination, the clinical psychologists tended to make use of what was already in their aramentarium;

the standard psychological tests.

While these two approaches never fully merged, the writings of
Goldstein and Scheerer (1941), and of Luria (1973), demonstrated
how clinical tests could be productively used in the assessment of
brain damaged patients. The Goldstein-Scheerer tests were probably
the first neuropsychological test battery used in the United States,
and although they are rarely used now in their original form, the
principles upon which they were established remain highly relevant
to construction of more modern instruments. For example, the loss
of the "abstract attitude," first systematically studied by Goldstein and Scheerer (1941) remains as a basic principle of impairment
of brain function, and neuropsychologists continue to use sorting
and categorizing tests, and other measures of abstraction, as parts
of their assessments.

While it was generally appreciated that specific clinical tests
were highly useful in the assessment of brain damaged patients, concern began to emerge involving the lack of standardization of these
procedures. There were no formal validity and reliability studies,
no norms or cut-off scores, and often no scoring system at all. As
it developed, at about the time Goldstein and Scheerer were conducting their investigations of abstract behavior, Ward Halstead was establishing what was perhaps the first human neuropsychology laboratory, at the University of Chicago. Halstead was an advocate of experimental methodology, the use of objective procedures with quantification and the practice of correlating behavioral deficits with
neurological evidence of the nature and location of brain damage.
Thus, he worked closely with a group of neurosurgeons in establishing a research program involving the development of laboratory procedures for detecting the consequences of lesions in various portions
of the brain, particularly the frontal lobes (Halstead, 1947). Halstead's student, Ralph Reitan, pursued the idea that these laboratory procedures, with some additions and modifications, could be used
productively in clinical assessment, both from practical and research
standpoints. The development of these procedures in the form of what
is now known as the Halstead-Reitan Neuropsychological Test Battery
(Reitan & Davison, 1974), takes us into the present; the modern era
of neuropsychological assessment.

The Halstead-Reitan Battery includes many of Halstead's original
discriminating tests, as well as a standard intelligence test (one
of the several Wechsler scales), the Trail Making test (Reitan, 1958)
and several additional measures of various language and perceptual
skills. It is the most widely used of the standard neuropsychological batteries, and has gained wide acceptance within American psychology. Nevertheless, not all clinical neuropsychologists have
accepted it. There are competing batteries, notably the Luria-
Nebraska Neuropsychological Test Battery (Golden, Hammeke & Purisch,
1980), but there are also those who do not advocate the use of a

fixed, standard battery at all. These neuropsychologists, such as
Benton (1982), and Lezak (1983), recommend a flexible approach, and
suggest that even though objective, standardized tests are desirable,
they should be used individually as appropriate for the assessment
of the individual patient being evaluated. The issue of "fixed" vs.
"flexible" testing remains as a major point of controversy in the
field (Goldstein, 1981).

It is probably fair to say that contemporary neuropsychological
assessment stands at a crossroad leading either to further developments along the quantitative, psychometrically oriented direction
pointed to by the Halstead-Reitan and Luria-Nebraska approaches, or
toward the more flexible, individualized approaches advocated by the
behavioral neurologists, notably Luria and his students, and those
clinical neuropsychologists who discourage the use of fixed, standard
batteries. It may be noted that Luria has recently been "rediscover-
ed," largely through the work of Christensen (1975), and many clinicians are now quite involved in using his method of neuropsychological investigation. This line of development should be dissociated,
however, from the Luria-Nebraska battery, which reflects a quantitative, psychometric approach, only utilizing test items used by Luria
in his qualitative, individualized examinations of patients.

Some Basic Principles of Neuropsychological Assessment

Following the neuropsychologist's administration of tests of
memory, intelligence, language and the other abilities discussed
above, the material obtained must be integrated in some manner. Obviously, such integration is to a great extent subjective in nature,
as is the case for essentially all forms of clinical assessment,
but even so, it must be based on some model of how the brain relates
to behavior. Earlier deliberations concerning how the brain functions tended to revolve around a debate between so-called localization theory in which the brain was seen as composed of a number of
centers for specific functions which are connected by associative
pathways and mass action or holistic theory, that postulated that the
brain always functions as an integrated whole. While this debate
was quite heuristic in the past, it now seems to be the case that
neither view in its extreme form is correct. Rather, the brain can
act in a localized or global manner, depending upon the nature of
the task it has to perform. Thus, brain damage of essentially
any type and in essentially any area, can give rise to both general
and specific effects. When the brain damaged patient is asked to
solve a complex cognitive task, such as forming a relatively difficult abstraction or solving a complex perceptual problem, impairment
may be noted, regardless of where the brain damage is localized.
However, the ability to perform a simple task, such as repeating a
word or identifying an object, is generally only impaired in patients
with structural damage to a particular region of the brain. Thus,

certain assessment instruments tap highly localizable functions,
while other instruments tap functions that tend to be impaired in
many, if not most, brain damaged patients.

It is also now well established that the two hemispheres of the
brain are different. In essentially all higher organisms, the nervous system is crossed such that the right brain controls the left
half of the body and vice versa. In humans, however, the brain is
functionally asymmetric with the right side mediating a number of
visual-spatial abilities and other nonverbal skills, while the left
side has to do with language. Thus, patients with aphasia and related language disorders frequently have sustained specific left
hemisphere brain damage and may have, in addition to the aphasia,
partial paralysis of the right side of the body. Patients having
difficulty with perceiving complex visual patterns (sometimes faces)
and constructing such patterns may have sustained right hemisphere
brain damage. Clinical neuropsychologists make extensive use of
this principle of functional asymmetry of the cerebral hemispheres
in their assessment work. The testing used to elicit evidence of
asymmetries is often found to be useful not only with regard to localization, but in determining the type of information processing
at which the patient may be defective. Thus, patients with left
hemisphere brain damage may have difficulties with analysis and sequential processing of information, while patients with right brain
damage may have their difficulties with simultaneous processing, or
the visual or auditory perception of patterns (Gazzaniga, 1970).

Most clinical neuropsychologists utilize the principle of hemisphere differences in two ways. They compare the right and left sides
of the body with various sensory and motor tasks, much like the neurologist examines for differences in sensation and reflexes between
the right and left side. They also, however, look at functional
asymmetries through administering various kinds of verbal and visual-
spatial tasks. In many patients, impairment in both cognitive and
sensory-motor domains are seen together, as in the case of the left
hemisphere stroke patient who is aphasic and partially paralyzed on
the right side, but sometimes only the cognitive asymmetries are
noted, or only the sensory-motor asymmetries. In relatively rare
cases, neither hemisphere in particular is defective, but the major
difficulty is with communication between the hemispheres. In these
disorders, known generally as callosal syndromes (Bogen, 1979), the
two hemispheres are disconnected by an act of nature, or through a
form of surgery used to treat intractable epilepsy known as cerebral
commisurotomy. The commisurotomy patient may demonstrate such phenomena as being unable to identify an object by touch when placed in
the left hand, but not when placed in the right hand. There is an
extensive literature concerning a series of these cases produced by
Roger Sperry and various collaborators (e.g., Sperry, Gazzaniga &
Bogen, 1969). Indeed, these cases have done much to refine our
knowledge of the differences between the two hemispheres.

The rather detailed information we have regarding hemisphere differences is not accompanied by an equivalent level of expertise concerning differences between the anterior and posterior portions of the brain. While it is known that the front of the brain has a great deal to do with the mediation of movement and the rear of the brain with the mediation of auditory, tactile and visual perception, neuropsychologists have not been generally successful in finding tests that distinguish well between patients with anterior and posterior lesions. While the frontal lobes have traditionally been an area of great neuropsychological interest, their specific functions remain far from fully understood. Luria (1973) has probably correctly pointed out that they have an important role in the formation of intentions, and in the planning and regulation of behavior, but not all authorities accept Luria's evidence for this view, although the general idea seems compatible with the observations of many clinicians. In general, however, most neuropsychologists would accept some notion of regional localization, recognizing that the frontal lobes mediate movement and perhaps certain higher functions, the occipital lobes vision, the temporal lobes hearing and the parietal lobes touch and other body senses. Obviously, the situation is much more complex than that, but we will only illustrate that point with some examples coming from the neurology of language and of memory.

Efforts are still underway to map out the language zone, particularly with the use of the CT scan (Naeser & Hayward, 1978). However, it now seems clear that a distinction may be made between so-called anterior and posterior aphasia. In anterior aphasia, speech is laborious and halting, and the lesion is in the fronto-temporal area of the left hemisphere. In posterior aphasia, speech is fluent but comprehension is poor. The responsible lesion is thought to be in the posterior portion of the left hemisphere. In some cases, the patient's aphasia is restricted to written language, and in this case the lesion is thought to be in the distribution of the left posterior cerebral artery. With regard to memory, there appear to be two major areas in the brain that are particularly crucial. Destruction of either of these areas can produce dense amnesia. One set of structures is the dorsomedial nucleus of the thalamus and the mammilary bodies. When these structures hemorrhage, the expected outcome is a Wernicke-Korsakoff encephalopathy which generally evolves into a Korsakoff's syndrome; a dense amnesia with particular impairment of recent memory. The other important structure is the hippocampus. The hippocampus is a structure deep in the temporal lobe, lying in the floor of the inferior horn of the lateral ventricle. It is a bilateral structure, with one in each hemisphere. Destruction of both hippocampi result in extremely dense, intractable amnesia that is distinguishable in some respects from the thalamic-mammilary body amnesias associated with Korsakoff syndrome. Basically, while Korsakoff syndrome is essentially an information processing defect having largely to do with degraded encoding of new

information, the hippocampal amnesias appear to simply involve a
failure to register new information.

The above material provides some examples of specific localization in contemporary neuropsychology. Thus, we have very non-
specific symptoms of brain damage, symptoms which are regionally
localizable, to the right or left hemisphere or to the anterior or
posterior portion of the brain, and symptoms which are specifically
localizable to particular structures. In retrospect, then, both
early localization and mass action theories, in their extreme forms,
did not do justice to the complexity of brain function, and did not
appreciate the point that the brain is capable of both highly integrated and highly differentiated functions.

Some Basic Principles of Neuropsychological Treatment

The chapters of this book by Drs. Helm-Estabrooks and Holland,
and by Drs. Stricker and Zigmond, each in their own way make a basic
point. Brain damage is not a static phenomenon; while many of the
brain disorders remain stable over many years, some of them get better and some get worse. This longitudinal aspect of brain function
is crucial for any discussion of treatment and rehabilitation. The
inability of central nervous system tissue to regenerate is well established, but the conclusions drawn from that fact have not always
been accurate. There is major recovery from many forms of brain
damage that is readily observed by anyone who has spent time on an
acute neurology or neurosurgery ward. In addition to the spontaneous recovery process, there seems to be sufficient plasticity in
brain function to allow for restoration of certain abilities as a
result of specific training. Drs. Helm-Estabrooks and Holland make
a good case for the view that this training often takes the patient
substantially beyond the natural recovery process. As neuropsychologists have begun working with brain damaged patients in rehabilitation settings, certain general principles have emerged, some of
which can be briefly summarized here.

First, as we have indicated, it would appear that treatment is
effective to an extent that surpasses what can be expected from natural recovery processes. This point has been documented by controlled group studies, and by studies of individual cases who were
treated long past the time when spontaneous recovery had taken its
course. Second, treatment can be maximally beneficial when it takes
advantage of the patient's residual capacities and detours around
areas of permanently impaired function. Certain goals can be reached
by a variety of routes, and it is generally important to avoid routes
that the patient can no longer use. Third, certain activities can
be improved by changing the level at which they are performed. Luria
(1963) refers to one aspect of this process as elevating the level of
the activity. Thus, for example, the patient who has difficulty

walking in a normal fashion may be helped by making walking into a
cognitive, rather than a habitual, activity. One method Luria used
to do this was to draw lines on the floor and have the patient step
on the lines. This addition of visual support and the making of the
task into a conscious effortful activity, rather than an automatic
habit, appeared to be associated with a remarkable improvement in
walking. Fourth, instructional methods used with brain damaged
patients must be appropriate to their diminished attentional and
information processing capacities. As Diller (1978) points out,
stimuli must be made more than usually salient, and it is often
necessary to break tasks down into incremental steps. Judicious use
must be made of cuing, and often it is necessary to help the patient
organize the material to be learned. For example, Cermak (1975) has
shown that Korsakoff patients remember better when they are taught
to encode stimuli by such means as organizing groups of words into
categories.

These considerations and others related to the particular characteristics of the patient's disorder, when properly applied, can
often be associated with substantial restoration of function in brain
damaged patients. While most patients clearly do not return to their
premorbid levels, they do acquire skills useful in ordinary activities of daily living and, to some extent, in vocational placement.
In working with brain damaged patients, the rehabilitative aspects
of the treatment program should be accompanied by a "case management"
component, in which the patient and the patient's family are guided
such that the patient is not prematurely exposed to situations with
which he cannot cope, or alternatively, not exposed to situations
which could be of therapeutic value.

The Place of Clinical Neuropsychology Among the Neurosciences and Neurological Disciplines

Neurology, as a broad field encompassing numerous subprofessions
and scientific disciplines, has made enormous strides during the past
two decades and each of its branches has had to reevaluate its role
relative to other branches. Perhaps the major challenge to clinical
neuropsychology came with the development of the CT scan, since it
became possible to visualize lesions that previously could often be
only identified indirectly through detailed clinical and behavioral
investigation. Up to the point of common use of the CT scan, neuropsychological testing compared quite favorably to other neurodiagnostic procedures. Perhaps the most well known study was accomplished
by Filskov and Goldstein (1974), who reported an accuracy level of
89% for neuropsychological tests, as compared with 80% for angiograms
and 16% for skull X-Rays. However, this investigation and those done
earlier did not involve the CT scan. Now we are beyond the CT scan,
and into measures of cerebral metabolism, such as positron emission
tomography (PET scan) and regional cerebral blood flow studies. The

new technique of nuclear magnetic resonance may take us even further
away from the venerable problem of the neurologist of being unable
to directly look at the organ that is his/her major interest. Thus,
it is becoming increasingly less frequent that clinical neuropsychological tests and other indirect procedures are called upon to
identify the presence and localization of brain lesions.

In view of these developments, it seems clear that recently neuropsychology has become less localization oriented and more concerned
with the specification of behavioral processes. However, it is also
becoming clear that the CT scan does not hold all of the answers to
problems posed in neurodiagnosis. While it clearly identifies atrophy and focal, structural lesions, such as infarcts or the effects
of trauma, there are many brain disorders that are not associated
with structural lesions and, thus, cannot be visualized by the CT
scan. Of course, as the technique develops, more and more can be
seen, but even so there will still be much that cannot be seen.
Thus, it is not uncommon to see patients with neuropsychological
deficits and a medical history consistent with some specific disorder, but with no abnormal findings on the CT scan. In some cases,
regional cerebral blood flow studies can identify pathology which
the CT scan does not identify (Buchsbaum & Ingvar, 1982). It would
now appear that being able to examine brain activity or metabolism
is often much more useful than simply visualizing structures.

In actuality, the development of the CT scan and related procedures appears to have had a salubrious influence on neuropsychology.
A major problem of the past has been that neuropsychological tests
often "ran ahead" of their criteria, so that while a diagnostic prediction may have been accurate, it could not be confirmed by physical evidence because of limitations in the diagnostic state of the
art at the time. Now with the CT scan and related procedures, it
has become increasingly possible to verify predictions made on the
basis of the neuropsychological assessment. Thus, such work as mapping out of the language zone mentioned above, can be carried out
with increasingly greater precision and sophistication. We may be
approaching the time when it might be possible to directly observe
brain activity during the course of ongoing behavior. Extremely interesting findings have come from correlating CT scan findings with
neuropsychological assessment, particularly in the areas of alcoholism (Hill & Mikhael, 1979), and schizophrenia (Weinberger & Wyatt,
1982). There are apparently meaningful associations between degree
of neuropsychological deficit and amount of neuronal depletion in
these cases. In general, then, the new brain imaging techniques
have ushered in a new, exciting era in clinical neuropsychology,
and rather than diminishing the relevance of the field, have really
provided it with the opportunity to significantly enhance its scientific basis.

A similar development has taken place with regard to neurosur-

gery. The use of the complete forebrain commisurotomy operation for
treatment of intractable epilepsy has led to many new insights concerning cerebral hemisphere asymmetries, with particular implications
for the role of language in human behavior (Gazzaniga, 1983). The
whole matter of "right hemisphere language" (Searleman, 1977) has
become a matter of active investigation again, primarily because of
the opportunity to examine each hemisphere separately in the split-
brain patients. These studies, in combination with studies of hem-
ispherectomy patients (Smith, 1981) have led to major new
developments in our understanding of hemisphere differences and
plasticity of brain function. It is particularly interesting to
note that several of the split-brain patients had their surgery many
years ago, and have developed adaptive mechanisms for dealing with
some of the cognitive and perceptual difficulties engendered by the
operation (Bogen, 1983). Future study of these adaptive mechanisms
will surely have important implications for rehabiliation and the
general understanding of adjustment to brain damage.

The impact of the discovery of the neurotransmitters and the
role of neuropeptides in brain functions on clinical neuropsychology
is not as yet clear. It seems established that the recovery immediately folloing brain insult is at least, in part, biochemically
mediated (Rubens, 1977), and that the etiology of many of the progressive neurological disorders, notably Alzheimer and Huntington
disease, are associated with primarily neurochemical disorders
(Boller et al., this volume). Those doing neurochemical and neuro-
pharmacological research have called upon neuropsychologists to
provide behavioral indices to assess the effects of their interven-
tions, particularly with regard to studies of compounds thought to
influence memory and learning abilities. Thus, neuropsychology has
found a relatively new role as a discipline collaborating with phar-
macologists, psychiatrists and neurologists with regard to the study
of substances that may in some way improve brain function (Growdon
& Corkin, 1980). While the results of these studies, thus far, have
been somewhat disappointing, it would seem worthwhile to take the
not yet accomplished step of combining administration of these new
drugs with the behavioral treatments established by rehabilitation
oriented neuropsychologists in order to determine the extent to
which there may be a synergistic effect not found when either form
of treatment is administered alone. It also seems possible that
the development of biochemical assay techniques for various neurological disorders may aid in the documentation of neuropsychological
test results. For example, efforts are underway to develop a laboratory technique for diagnosis of Huntington disease in vulnerable
individuals, even before the early symptoms appear. The related
field of genetics is also becoming a matter of interest to neuropsychologists, and there are the beginnings of research involving
the study of families. For example, it was recently reported
(Parsons, personal communication) that there is a greater degree of
neuropsychological deficit in nonalcoholics who had a positive

family history of alcoholism than in nonalcoholics without such a
family history.

In summary, clinical neuropsychology appears to be becoming an
increasingly interdisciplinary field, and members of the profession
are actively collaborating with surgeons, radiologists, pharmacolo-
gists and psychiatrists, in addition to their more traditional collaboration with neurologists and neurosurgeons. Advances in neuro-
radiology and neurochemistry have had major impacts on the field,
and neuropsychological research has begun to tie-in with developments
in these areas, particularly with regard to the CT scan and related
procedures, and to the development of the new learning and memory
enhancing drugs. There also appears to be an increasing amount of
interaction with the health professions in general. Neuropsychologists are working with internists and other medical specialists in
such areas as diabetes, hypertension, pulmonary disease, and the
effects of environmental pollutants. There appears to be increasing
awareness that brain function is, to a great extent, dependent on
health status in general, and that many "non-neurological" disorders
may have important implications for neuropsychological status.

Future Directions

While the topics for future volumes of this series have not been
selected yet, except for the next volume which will be concerned with
child neuropsychology, the material offered here might well suggest
certain directions in which to proceed. As we have indicated, it is
our feeling that the field is becoming increasingly concerned with
process and with treatment, and decreasingly concerned with the use
of neuropsychological tests in localization of brain lesions. It
also appears that some neuropsychologists have extended their interests into three areas: psychiatric patients, patients with illnesses
other than neurological diseases, and neuropsychological functioning
in normal individuals. Within neuropsychology's more traditional
area, there is increasing interest in the CT scan and related imaging techniques, particularly with regard to correlating quantitative
indices derived from these methods with behavioral data. Such major
programs as mapping out the language zone through use of the CT scan
and determining the degree of association between density or atrophy
measurements and degree of dementia are now underway. There are some
puzzling findings concerning the lack of correspondence between atrophy and dementia which need to be resolved (Boller et al., this volume), and there is, of course, the more general, significant problem
of "nonstructural" lesions that will probably never be seen by even
the most sophisticated imaging technique, except perhaps by those
methods that measure brain metabolism.

With regard to the matter of process, it would not be difficult
to imagine an entire volume devoted to the neuropsychology of memory,

language, spatial relations, or learning. Within each of these
areas, there is ample opportunity for even more detailed consideration, such as specific consideration of short-term memory or language comprehension. The basic question in all of these areas relates
to how the brain mediates the particular process. How is language
or three-dimensional space represented in the brain? What changes
take place in the brain as a result of learning? Neuropsychologists
have tended to answer questions of this type through studying marker
cases of patients with lesions of particular locations. It is now
possible to do more of this because of the new imaging techniques,
and it is probably no longer necessary to restrict this type of investigation largely to patients who have had surgery or who have come
to autopsy.

Many neuropsychologists are very concerned with specific populations, and it is also possible to organize material along that
line. Several chapters of this volume are devoted to special populations: aphasic, amnesic and psychiatric patients, and patients
with Alzheimer disease and related dementias. Other populations
certainly come to mind: children with learning disabilities, epileptics, patients with multiple sclerosis and related disorders,
head injured patients, and so on. Less extensively treated, but
of great current interest, would be populations of individuals who
have experienced malnutrition, excessive exposure to environmental
pollutants or who have systemic disorders with implications for
brain function such as diabetes, hypertension or chronic obstructive
pulmonary disease.

With regard to the matters of treatment and rehabilitation,
there is particularly great activity in that area, and much is already known about the efficacies of various pharmacological agents,
as well as various forms of behavioral treatment. As indicated,
neuropsychologists are involved in this work at several levels,
either as evaluators of the efficacy of treatment or as innovators
and evaluators of the treatments themselves. There is a revival of
interest in the way in which Luria (1963) approached the problem of
treatment and rehabilitation, and there are several centers now
active in doing treatment, as well as in educating the professional
public regarding what they do. The group at the NYU Institute of
Rehabilitation Medicine under the leadership of Leonard Diller is
notable in this regard.

It is apparent that there are many more topics than there are
possible volumes for this series, and we only can suggest a number
of possibilities. It is likewise apparent that the field of neuropsychology is rapidly expanding, and any attempt to produce an annual or bi-annual report on advances in the field must of necessity
be highly selective. In view of this wide range of possibilities,
we may at least point out what we do not propose to do. In particular, we will not devote a volume of the series to any particular

procedure, such as a particular neuropsychological test battery,
a particular treatment method or philosophy or some specialized
neurodiagnostic technique. Rather, we will attempt to continue
to have clinicians, clinical researchers and basic scientists contribute to selected areas of general interest which constitutes
some focus of major concern to the discipline of clinical neuropsychology as a whole.

References

Benton, A., 1982, Discussion - Symposium: Luria-Nebraska/Halstead-
    Reitan research with children and adolescents. Annual meeting
    of the American Psychological Association, Washington, D.C.
Bogen, J. E., 1979, The callosal syndrome, in: "Clinical Neuropsycho-
    logy," K. Heilman and E. Valenstein, eds., Oxford University
    Press, New York.
Bogen, J. E., 1983, A systematic quantitative study of cross-
    retrieval in long term follow-up of commisurotomy, Lecture
    presented at Western Psychiatric Institute and Clinic, Pitts-
    burgh, PA.
Boller, F., Goldstein, G., Gore, C., Kim, Y., Richey, E. T., Wagner,
    D. and Wolfson, S., In Press, Alzheimer and related dementias: A
    review of current knowledge, in: "Advances in Clinical Neuro-
    psychology, Vol. 1," G. Goldstein, ed., Plenum Press, New York.
Broca, P., 1861, Nouvelle observation d'aphemie produite par une
    lesion de la moite posterieure des deusieme et troisieme
    circonvolutions frontales, Societé Anatomique de Paris, 36:398-
    407.
Buchsbaum, M. S. and Ingvar, D. H., 1982, New visions of the schizo-
    phrenic brain: Regional differences in electrophysiology, blood
    flow, and cerebral glucose use, in: "Schizophrenia as a Brain
    Disease," F. A. Henn and H. A. Nasrallah, eds., Oxford University
    Press, New York.
Butters, N. and Cermak, L. S., 1980, "Alcoholic Korsakoff's Syndrome"
    Academic Press, New York.
Cermak, L. S., 1975, Imagery as an aid to retrieval for Korsakoff
    patients, Cortex, 11:163-169.
Christensen, A.-L., 1975, "Luria's Neuropsychological Investigation,"
    Spectrum Publications, New York.
Diller, L., 1976, A model for cognitive retraining in rehabilitation,
    The Clin. Psychol., 29:13-15.
Ferris, S. H., Reisberg, B., Crook, T., Friedman, E., Schneck, M. K.,
    Mir, P., Sherman, K. A., Corwin, J., Gershon, S., and Bartus, R.
    T., 1982, Pharmacologic treatment of senile dementia: Choline
    l-dopa, piracetam, and choline plus piracetam, in: "Alzheimer's
    Disease: A Review of Progress, Raven Press, New York.
Filskov, S. B. and Goldstein, S. G., 1974, Diagnostic validity of the
    Halstead-Reitan neuropsychological battery, J. Consult. Clin.
    Psychol., 42:382-388.

Gazzaniga, M. S., 1970, "The Bisected Brain", Appleton-Century-Crofts, New York.

Gazzaniga, M. S., 1983, Right hemisphere language following brain bisection: A 20-year perspective, Am. Psychol., 38:525-537.

Golden, C. J., Hammeke, T. A. and Purisch, A. D., 1980, "The Luria-Nebraska Battery Manual," Western Psychological Services, California.

Goldstein, G., 1981, Some recent developments in clinical neuropsychology, Clin. Psychol. Rev., 1:245-268.

Goldstein, G. and Neuringer, C., 1976, "Empirical Studies of Alcoholism," Ballinger, Cambridge, Massachusetts.

Goldstein, G. and Ruthven, L., 1983, "Rehabilitation of the Brain-Damaged Adult," Plenum, New York.

Goldstein, G. and Shelly, C.H., 1974, Neuropsychological diagnosis of multiple sclerosis in a psychiatric setting, J. Nerv. Ment. Dis, 158:280-290.

Goldstein, K. and Scheerer, M. Abstract and concrete behavior: An experiemental study with special tests, Psychol. Mono., 53:239.

Goodglass, H. and Kaplan, E., 1972, "The Assessment of Aphasia and Related Disorders," Lea and Febiger, Philadelphia, PA.

Growdon, J. H. and Corkin, S. Neurochemical approaches to the treatment of senile dementia, in: "Psychopathology in the Aged," J. O. Cole and J. E. Barrett, Raven Press, New York.

Gruzelier, J. and Flor-Henry, P., 1979, "Hemisphere Asymmetries of Function in Psychopathology", Elsevier/North-Holland, Amsterdam.

Halstead, W. C., 1947, "Brain and Intelligence," University of Chicago Press, Chicago.

Heaton, R. K. and Crowley, T. J., 1981, Effects of psychiatric disorders and their somatic treatments on neuropsychological test results, in "Handbook of Clinical Neuropsychology," T. J. Boll and S. B. Filskov, eds., Wiley-Interscience, New York.

Henn, F. A. and Nasrallah, H. A., 1982, "Schizophrenia as a Brain Disease, Oxford University Press, New York.

Hill, S. Y. and Mikhael, M., 1979, Computerized transaxical and tomographic and neuropsychological evaluation in chronic alcoholics and heroin abusers, Am. J. Psych., 136:598-602.

Kertesz, A., 1979, "Aphasia and Associated Disorders: Taxonomy, Localization and Recovery," Grune and Stratton, New York.

Kimura, D. and Durnford, M., 1974, Normal studies on the function of the right hemisphere in vision, in: "Hemisphere Function in the Human Brain", S. J. Dimond and J. G. Beaumont, eds., Elek Science, London.

Lezak, M. D., 1976, "Neuropsychological Assessment," Oxford University Press, New York.

Luria, A. R., 1963, "Restoration of Function After Brain Injury," MacMillan, New York.

Luria, A. R., 1973, "The Working Brain," Basic Books, New York.

Naeser, M. A. and Hayward, R. W., 1978, Lesion localization in aphasia with cranial computed tomography and the Boston Diagnostic Aphasia Exam, Neurology, 28:545-551.

Reisberg, B., Ferris, S. H. and Gershon, S., 1980, Pharmacotherapy of
    senile dementia, in: "Psychopathology in the Aged," J. O. Cole
    and J. E. Barrett, eds., Raven Press, New York.
Reitan, R. M., 1958, Validity of the trail making test as an
    indicator of organic brain damage, Percept. Mot. Skills, 8:271-
    276.
Reitan, R. M. and Davison, L. A., 1974, "Clinical Neuropsychology:
    Current Status and Applications", V. H. Winston, Washington, D.C.
Ross, A. T. and Reitan, R. M., 1955, Intellectual and affective
    functions in multiple sclerosis: A quantitative study, Arch.,
    Neuro. Psych., 73:663-677.
Rubens, A., 1977, The role of changes within the central nervous
    system during recovery from aphasia, in: "Rationale for Adult
    Aphasia Therapy," M. Sullivan and M. Kommens, eds., University of
    Nebraska Press, Omaha.
Searleman, A., 1977, A review of right hemisphere linguistic
    capabilities, Psychol. Bull., 84:503-528.
Smith, A., 1981, Principles underlying human functions in neuro-
    psychological sequelae of different neuropathological processes,
    in: "Handbook of Clinical Neuropsychology," S. B. Filskov and T.
    J. Boll, eds., Wiley-Interscience, New York.
Sperry, R. W., Gazzaniga, M. S. and Bogen, J. E., 1969, Inter-
    hemispheric relationships: The neocortical commisures; syndromes
    of hemisphere disconnection, in: "Handbook of Clinical Neurology"
    P. J. Vinkin and G. W. Bruyen, eds., North Holland, Amsterdam.
Teuber, H. -L., 1959, Some alterations in behavior after cerebral
    lesions in man, in: "Evolution of Nervous Control from Primitive
    Organisms to Man," A. D. Bass, ed., American Association for the
    Advancement of Science, Washington, D.C.
Weinberger, D. R. and Wyatt, R. J., 1982, Brain morphology in
    schizophrenia, in: "Schizophrenia as a Brain Disease," F. A.
    Henn and H. A. Nasrallah, eds., Oxford University Press, New
    York.

RECENT DEVELOPMENTS IN CLINICAL NEUROPSYCHOLOGY

Oscar A. Parsons

Department of Psychiatry and Behavioral Sciences
University of Oklahoma Health Sciences Center
Oklahoma City, Oklahoma

Over a decade ago, I completed a survey of clinical neuropsychology which I described as a new, emergent speciality in clinical
psychology. The paper was published in 1970 (Parsons, 1970) in a
rather "off-the-beaten-path" (for neuropsychologists) series, "Current Topics in Clinical and Community Psychology." The present chapter can be seen as constituting an evaluation of how this assessment
has held up.

The essential points made in the 1970 chapter were as follows.
In the section entitled, "Clinical Neuropsychology: a New Discipline,"
I defined clinical neuropsychology as "that branch of psychology
which applies knowledge derived from relevant experimental and clinical investigations to specific brain-behavior problems in humans."
I noted that the clinical neuropsychologist is concerned primarily
with identifying, measuring and describing changes in behavior that
relate to brain dysfunction. Thus, the clinical neuropsychologist's
activities contribute to a variety of important clinical problems:
differential diagnosis; lateralization and localization of lesions;
establishing baselines of sensory, motor, perceptual, cognitive and
intellectual functioning from which subsequent improvement or decline
can be determined; identifying specific deficits from noxious agents
such as drugs; developing methods for remediation of deficit; help-
ing to determine competency in the aged; and, developing better diagnostic and remedial efforts for the minimally brain-damaged child.

I predicted that these specific functions would grow in importance in that the society in which we live is one "whose youth ex-
periments with multifarious mind (brain) altering drugs, whose over-
thirty population is ridden with alcohol and tranquilizers, whose
underprivileged frequently suffer from inadequate diets which

19

directly in the neonate or indirectly in a pregnant mother affect
the growing brain, and whose automobile drivers provide a toll of
head injuries from accidents that outstrips wartime casualties."

Certainly the prediction of the growth of clinical neuropsychology has been borne out, even more so, I believe, than had been
originally emphasized or envisioned. Journals such as Neuropsychologia and Cortex have survived their adolescence and settled into
competent maturity; Brain and Language seems to be well established
and two new journals, Clinical Neuropsychology and the Journal of
Clinical Neuropsychology have recently been started. In our most
prestigious scientific journal, Science, papers on neuropsychology
regularly appear. There has been a spate of new texts; where for
several years we had only Luria's Higher Cortical Functions in Man
(1966), Russell, Neuringer and Goldstein's Assessment of Brain Damage (1970), and Small's Neuropsychodiagnosis and Psychotherapy (1973),
we have seen Reitan and Davison's Clinical Neuropsychology (1974),
Lezak's Neuropsychological Assessment (1976), Golden's Diagnosis and
Rehabilitation in Clinical Neuropsychology (1978), Hecaen and Albert's
Human Neuropsychology (1978), Walsh's Neuropsychology: A clinical
approach (1978), and the latest arrival, Heilman and Valenstein's
Clinical Neuropsychology (1979). There are at least three books
close to publication of which I am aware; undoubtedly there are
others.

As a reviewer for papers on neuropsychology in one of our most
widely read clinical psychological journals, the Journal of Consulting and Clinical Psychology, I can attest to the fact that neuropsychological papers are being submitted at an unprecedented rate.
As a member of the Veteran's Administration National Merit Review
Committee in the Behavioral Sciences, I have been amazed at the number of projects involving neuropsychological measurement throughout
the VA system. Out of the 13-member Board, we have 3 neuropsychologists and could use another in these grant application reviews.

The International Neuropsychological Society has grown from a
rather informal, low-key, semi-organized group to a flourishing
society which has meetings of quality both in the United States and
abroad. The membership is now over one thousand. We have just
created a Division of Clinical Neuropsychology in the American Psychological Association; it will certainly call even greater attention
to the specialized contributions of our field. A special interest
group in Behavioral Neuropsychology has been formed within the Association for the Advancement of Behavior Therapy (Horton, 1979). The
1979 APA program in New York had the greatest number of explicitly
designated sessions on neuropsychological problems it has ever had
and subsequent APA programs have contained extensive contributions
from neuropsychology. Workshops in neuropsychology have become
commonplace; indeed, we find that they have really achieved status
when you can enroll in such a workshop while on a Carribean Cruise!

What factors are responsible for this amazing growth? I believe that there are at least five potent influences. First, the explosion in number of basic neuroscience investigations at neurobehavioral and neuroanatomic levels has created a pool of exciting new information, much of which has potential applied value. Communication of these findings to the scientific world and the interested citizen provides constant stimulus; that is, the September, 1979, issue of Scientific American was devoted in its entirety to the brain. Second, specific technological advances in human biomedical brain techniques such as computed tomography (CT), cerebral blood flow quantification, event-related potentials and EEG quantification have provided new and effective criterion measures to which behavioral change can be related. Third, advances in psychological theory such as information processing, decision making, memory and other cognitive processes have provided new avenues of exploration for neuropsychology. Fourth, the advent of low cost microprocessors and computers has enabled neuropsychologists to apply multivariate statistics to a variety of problems with heuristic and comprehensive outcomes. Finally, there are specific contributions from neuropsychologists, themselves, who have gained the respect of other colleagues by their substantive efforts in the field.

What has been achieved? In subsequent sections of this paper, I shall consider recent progress in neuropsychological assessment, rehabilitation and retraining, and finally, research on hemispheric asymmetries. Space constraints are such that I must be quite selective; the coverage obviously is biased - one person's view of important developments. With that restriction in mind, let us consider some recent developments in our field.

Clinical Neuropsychological Assessment

While the growth of clinical neuropsychology is attributable to a variety of factors, in my opinion, the preeminent spur has been the prodigious work of Ralph Reitan, with the Halstead Battery (Reitan & Davison, 1974). Indeed, in recognition of his contributions, most workers in the field refer to the Battery now as the "Halstead-Reitan Battery" (HRB). I need not detail the particulars of the developments of the HRB, as they are readily available in numerous sources (Reitan & Davison, 1974). I should point out several major facts. Halstead (1947) originally developed the Battery by attempting to derive a number of measures of "biological intelligence" rather than "psychometric intelligence." The former was to be a measure of the organism's adaptability to life rather than reflecting educational experiences, as in many intelligence tests. Halstead empirically selected those tests which gave rise to the best discrimination between brain-damaged and nonbrain-damaged subjects. He attempted to order the tests through factor analysis and arrive at a theoretical conception of "biological intelligence." While his theorizing has never had much impact, the empirical find-

ings have been remarkable. Reitan and his colleagues' work provided
quantification, standardization and validity for the tests (Boll,
1978; Reitan, & Davison, 1974). Their demonstration of the Battery's
ability to detect damage, lateralize and localize lesions; their scientific productivity - many studies with large numbers of brain-damaged patients; the extension of the Battery to children; the demonstration of the relationship of selected aspects of the Battery with
other biomedical techniques such as the EEG - all produced a substantive body of knowledge that gave clinical neuropsychology a firm
base from which to work, as well as a base which captured attention
and respect from neurologists, neurosurgeons, psychiatrists, peer
psychologists, and other health professionals.

The HRB received further impetus with the publication in 1970
by Russell, Neuringer and Goldstein of their "neuropsychological key"
approach. These investigators described a systematic decision-making
process in which the application of quantitative indices derived from
the HRB results in statements as to presence or absence of brain damage; severity of damage; lateralized or diffuse-if lateralized which
side and whether weakly or strongly lateralized; and finally, whether
the damage is acute, congenital or static. The system lends itself
well to computer programming and analysis. Thus, entry of the data
gives a computer print-out with statements similar to those described
above. In the decade following the publication of their monograph,
there has been a steady growth in the number of laboratories who have
adopted their method of scoring and analysis of the HRB. Golden
(1977) has recently presented additional data confirming the utility
of the Key approach. Aaron (1979) has adopted their approach to develop a systematic deductive procedure for the diagnosis and remediation of learning disabilities, although tests other than the HRB
are employed.

The latest development in HRB research, appropriately enough,
has come from Reitan and is directed toward children. Selz and
Reitan (1979) have developed rules for neuropsychological diagnosis
based on a quantification of Reitan's four methods of inference;
that is, level of performance, right-left differences, patterns
(variability) of performance and pathognomonic signs. Application
of 37 rules enabled classification of children from 9-14 into three
groups; normal, learning disability or brain damaged, with 73% accuracy. The importance of this presentation lies in its specification of the rules and their application on a quantified basis; thus
making explicit what has heretofore been judgmental and imprecise.

It seems to me that with the development of these rules, the
limits of the development of the HRB have been reached. The con-
ribution to clinical neuropsychology has been, is, and will be enormous. The HRB epitomizes much of the quantitative approach to psychology in the United States. In using the HRB, empirical data have
been generated which not only have differentiated brain-damaged and

nonbrain-damaged persons, but allowed discriminating statements to
be made by experienced neuropsychologists concerning the extent,
severity, location, lateralization, nature and progress of the lesion.
However, in my opinion, the ultimate limiting factor, the lack of a
neuropsychological model or theory, will preclude any further development other than modest refinements.

If a neuropsychological theory or model is deemed desirable,
to whom do we turn? The late Russian neuropsychologist, Alexander
Luria, is the obvious candidate. Luria's work over the last several
decades (Luria, 1966; Luria & Majovski, 1977), provided us with a
thorough and detailed working model of neuropsychological functioning. In brief, Luria considers the brain as comprised of a series
of functional systems contributing to the whole of the functioning.
It is also characterized by "functional pluripotentialism," which
means that a given system's function can be taken over by other functional systems. The fact that a given deficit occurs in perception,
memory or other higher cortical functions is not the end of the psychological assessment but from Luria's point of view, the beginning
of the problem. Each symptom is analyzed by a variety of different
techniques in order to determine which factors are important in the
disturbed behavior. Consequently, the reliance is upon individually
administered tests by a highly skilled professional. As Luria points
out, testing is never to be construed (as it may be in the case of
the HRB) as the mechanistic application of a standardized test battery with a formal quantitative interpretation of the results. In
contradistinction, it is a "clinically creative effort requiring
from the neuropsychologist both critical thinking and readiness to
reject initial hypotheses when they conflict with new data obtained"
(Luria & Majovski, 1977). Thus, the examiner has a variety of techniques and, dependent upon the immediate performance of the patient,
pursues different courses. Of course, this method is decidedly different from the HRB approach in the hands of Reitan and his students
or in the modifications introduced by the Key approach.

Luria's theory is persuasive and his case illustrations are always very instructive. However, the lack of quantification of his
tests, and particularly the lack of norms which define how good or
bad the person is performing, means that only individuals highly
trained by Luria or his colleagues can really administer the tests
effectively - a situation which American neuropsychologists cannot
tolerate. In February of 1978, in a talk on the past, present and
future of neuropsychology, I concluded my talk with:

> Finally, I believe that we will see the devel-
> opment of neuropsychological theory to a greater
> extent during the next decade. The question is,
> will Luria's theory be like that of Piaget - pro-
> vocative, insightful and helpful as a general
> orientation, but not particularly helpful in

dealing with specific behavioral measures, or
will the promise of Luria's claims be realized
in the form of specific behavioral measures
for diagnosis, identification of deficits and
remediation of them? Will there, in other words,
be a Reitan for Luria as there was for Halstead?
My answer is yes, I believe that by 1990 we will
have a Luria Battery equivalent to the Halstead
Battery of the day (Parsons, 1978).

My prediction was correct in one respect; we have had a quantification of the Luria Battery, but ten years earlier than I expected.
Charles Golden and his associates at the University of South Dakota,
and more recently at the University of Nebraska Medical Center, have
developed this quantification in an energetic, comprehensive and
sophisticated manner. Using the rich insights of Luria in his many
books and articles, and the clinical manuals for the Luria techniques
developed by Anne-Lise Christensen (1975a, 1975b), Golden et al.
(1978; Golden, 1979) have provided a scaling of the eleven dimensions
of higher cortical functioning formulated by Christensen and Luria;
conducted validation and cross-validation studies discriminating
brain-damaged from controls; compared brain-damage and schizophrenic
populations with the Luria discriminating brain-damaged from schizophrenics at a fairly high level (Purisch, Golden, & Hammeke, 1978);
found mild but significant impairment in alcoholics; found ventricular enlargement as measured by CT scan to be significantly related
to impaired Luria scoring in both schizophrenic and alcoholic populations; demonstrated that lateralization and localization of functions could be achieved by discriminant function analysis; factor-
analyzed the various primary scales; developed corrections for age
and education; provided guidelines for interpretation of findings;
and, currently are developing a children's version (Golden, 1978;
Golden, 1981).

The Luria Standardized Battery has a number of advantages: a
skilled and experienced tester can halve the time required for the
HRB; scores are obtained for eleven primary functions: motor, acous-
ticomotor, cutaneous and kinesthetic, visual, impressive speech,
expressive speech, reading, writing, artithmetic, mnestic processes,
intellectual processes, and for three additional scales; a patho-
gnomic scale (items which appear to best discriminate brain-damaged
from controls) and a "left hemisphere" scale and a "right hemisphere"
scale (based mainly on sensorimotor performance). Again, and perhaps most importantly, the operations are tied to a neuropsychological theory, thus laying the groundwork for rehabilitation and retraining. While the application of the Luria Standardized Battery
is in its infancy, it is already clear that the potential is great.
My prediction is that the next decade will see the flourishing of
the Luria Battery in the same way that the HRB flowered over the last
decade.

It is inevitable that comparisons between the HRB and the Luria Standardized Battery be made. In the first comparison of the two batteries, Kane, Moses and Sweet (1979) had two experienced neuropsychologists rate brain-damaged and nonbrain-damaged psychiatric (including schizophrenics!) patients as brain-damaged or not brain-damaged from the summary scores of the HRB; if brain-damaged, the cases were next rated as to whether the major brain damage was in the right hemisphere, the left hemisphere, or bilateral diffuse. One neuropsychologist (the present author) made the ratings on the basis of the HRB. The other judge (Dr. Charles Golden), experienced in the Luria Standardized Battery, made the same ratings on the basis of the Luria scores. Overall identification of brain-damaged versus nonbrain-damaged, was approximately the same; approximately 80% for each and the two raters agreed on approximately 82% of the cases.

As regards lateralization, left hemisphere and right hemisphere cases were correctly identified at about the same level, but the HRB rater called more of the diffuse-bilateral cases right hemisphere. While this study must be regarded as quite preliminary, and in obvious need of extension to more raters other than the two used, we can be impressed by the congruence of the data.

Will the Luria Battery prove useful with children and aged adults? These two populations pose special problems in neuropsychological assessment. I have already noted two such approaches with children, one by Selz and Reitan (1979), based on the HRB, and one by Aaron (1979), using the Key approach. Sollee and collaborators (1979), in their recent APA symposium, exemplified the use of a neuropsychological approach to brain-damaged children and their rehabilitation by emphasizing qualitative as well as quantitative approaches. In discussing the Symposium presentations, Edith Kaplan forcefully brought home the importance of measuring the way the patient attempts the task as well as the end product. Her description of differences in right, left, and frontal-damaged patients' approaches to performance on the Block Design highlighted her point. More work of this nature is urgently needed.

The problems of assessment of the elderly are receiving increasing attention. There is no question about the fact that there is an increasing percentage of the population over the age of 65. With greater logevity has come an increase in the senile and pre-senile dementias. The standard neuropsychological tests, such as the HRB, are much too long and probably too difficult (e.g., the Category and TPT tests) for the older person. Kazniak, Kelly, and Schneider (1978) have constructed a short battery (90 minutes) which relies on items (thought to be discriminating for brain dysfunction) taken from various widely used psychological tests and, hence, readily available to most psychologists. They also tried to get a broad sampling of mental abilities thought to be important in aging, such as language skills, writing, reading, motor functions, recent and remote memory and other tests from which one could infer differential impairment of lateralized functions.

Test-retest reliability of their battery was high. To assess validity, a neurologically normal aged group was compared to a group with neurological evidence of brain dysfunction. The groups differed on all but one of 16 comparisons and with discriminant function analyses, 95% were diagnosed correctly. Further, right and left hemisphere patients could be distinguished reliably. Finally, modest but significant correlations of many of the subtests with CT measures of atrophy and EEG slowing have been found. This Battery has obviously been carefully constructed and will undoubtedly receive a great deal of attention in the future.

Regardless of neuropsychological assessment procedures used, it seems safe to say that these procedures will become used more rather than less during the years ahead. The increasingly important role that neuropsychological assessment occupies with patients for whom there is compensation and/or litigation involved, has raised some interesting issues. In one of the most provocative studies of this decade, Robert Heaton at the University of Colorado College of Medicine (Heaton, Smith, Lehman, & Vogt, 1978) had individuals feign a history of head trauma. They were given certain types of vague symtoms to report and a case history "cover" but were given no other instructions as to how to behave on the HRB other than perform as they thought patients might perform if head-injured. Technicians, naive with respect to the study, administered the tests in the standard HRB fashion, to both these subjects and actual head-injured cases.

Disconcerting results were obtained: the malingerers and actual head-injured did not differ significantly on their overall level of neuropsychological performance. However, there were different patterns of strengths and deficits produced by the two groups on testing. It is interesting that on some tests the malingerers did much more poorly (e.g., sensory-motor tests) than the head-injured, whereas on some others (e.g., TPT, Categories) they did better. The protocols were sent to ten neuropsychologists who were recognized as competent to make "blind" judgments as to whether each protocol was produced by a malingerer or by a real head-injury patient. The results ranged from near chance to modestly better than chance. Application of a discriminant function analysis plus the MMPI correctly classified 94% of the subjects. Heaton and his collaborators then applied this procedure to another sample of head-injury patients who were involved in court action with a group of similar patients who were not so involved. There were 42 patients in each group. Sixty-four percent of the former were classified as being malingerers by the discriminant function formula, compared with 26% of the latter. Obviously, this study raises important issues and should receive the close attention of all practicing neuropsychologists.

Retraining and Rehabilitation

It is interesting that clinical neuropsychology has only relatively recently emphasized rehabilitation (Parsons & Prigatano,
1978). Kurt Goldstein's After-Effects of Brain Injury in War, published in English in 1942 (but covering work done in the early
1920s), provided an extensive discussion of various rehabilitative
approaches of a psychological, educational, work sample, sociofamil-
ial nature in rehabilitating brain-damaged persons. His book can be
read today with as much profit as it was originally. Why has there
been the benign neglect of his work? Probably because Goldstein's
approach was very much that of the skilled clinician. While he used
quantitative data, he was much more interested in qualitative observations as they related to his concept of abstract vs. concrete at-
titudes. These concepts could not be easily quantified as required
by our typical American tradition and, therefore, norms for such
behaviors were lacking. However, in order to rehabilitate or retrain,
one must have some type of quantitative measure from which to judge
progress - even though the quantification my be ordinal.

As psychology proper and neuropsychology in particular have developed quantitative procedures and methods, the bases for measuring
change have been established. Concomitantly, there has been a rise
in behaviorally and cognitively behaviorally-oriented educational
techniques for effecting behavioral change (Goldstein, 1979). Finally, the emphasis by Luria (1966) on capacity of the human brain to
reorganize and adapt to a change in structure, so that given "functions in behavior" may be achieved by different brain systems, has
encouraged us to think along rehabilitative lines. Indeed, Luria's
1969 chapter on the topic of "restoration of higher cortical functions following local brain damage" is another classic which demands
periodic re-reading.

During the 1970s, then, there has been an increasing interest
in retraining and rehabilitation by neuropsychologists. The programs
of Leonard Diller and Yehuda Ben-Yishay at the Institute of Rehabilitation Medicine, New York University Medical Center, are notable in
this regard. In 1979, the 7th annual workshop on remediation of cognitive deficits in brain damage was conducted under the leadership of
these psychologists. Their methods and approaches to this type of
rehabilitation are detailed in supplements for the workshop (Ben-
Yishay, 1978, 1979). It is quite evident that the rehabilitation
process demands a high level of knowledge, skill, inventiveness, per-
sistence and motivation in the re-trainer or therapist.

On the West Coast, Lewinsohn and his colleagues (1977) at the
University of Oregon, have conducted an extensive investigation of
assessment and remediation of memory deficits in brain-damaged patients. In one study, they used visual imagery training techniques
in conjunction with a paired associate learning and a face name

learning task. On both tasks, the treatment had its desired effect
in both controls and brain-damaged; that is, a marked improvement
occurred when tested 30 minutes after acquisition. However, one
week later, neither the patients nor the controls manifested savings
from the imagery training!

Work with individuals in Lewinsohn's laboratories on a case-by-
case basis has been somewhat more successful. Glasgow, Zeiss, Barrera, and Lewinsohn (1977) describe two patients in whom visual imagery techniques seemed to help a good deal in recovery of memory
functions. These patients were both in their early twenties, as
compared with Lewinsohn's previous study where the average patient
age was 42. Age is probably a very important variable in retraining
memory. These and other results lead Lewinsohn, Danaher, and Kikel
(1977) to comment:

> ...we suggest that effective interventions
> will probably require a synthesis of the
> knowledge in educational psychology, exper-
> imental psychology, neuropsychology, clinical
> psychology (especially behavioral self-control
> procedures) and the historical tradition of
> the early mnemonists...

While the focus of much of current discussion of rehabilitation
is upon cognitive-perceptual retraining, workers who have spent time
in the field agree that the patient's pre-morbid personality pattern
of strengths and weaknesses and their emotional response to their
changed abilities, play an important role in outcome. Prigatano
(1977) reported on serial measures of recovery of a young man seriously brain-injured at age 21 until the age of 27. While the patient
recovered to an average range of intelligence and had a Halstead-
Reitan Battery Impairment Index within the normal range, he had a
verbal handicap and slowness which hampered his social interaction.
He remained unhappy and socially isolated.

The importance of the interpersonal aspects of the patient who
has suffered brain damage is emphasized in another patient seen in
our laboratory. This patient was a 32-year-old married man who had
suffered an arteriovenous malformation on the left side for which he
was successfully operated. While there was residual neuropsychological deficit, he was able to return to his work as a carpenter. He
complained of depressive feelings and low self-esteem. When seen by
one of our postdoctorals, it became apparent that the marriage was
foundering, the couple had not had sexual relationships since the
brain operation, although there was no physical basis for the patient's lack of potency. A therapeutic program was devised which
first focused upon communication in the marriage and second, upon
a graded series of pleasuring techniques (following Masters & Johnson). After approximately five weeks, communication had improved

markedly and normal marital relationships were resumed; work adjustment was better.

It was clear that before the brain dysfunction the marriage had
been in trouble; the difficulties were enhanced by the patient's feeling of loss of ability, lowered self-esteem and depression. Therapy
considered not only the loss of neuropsychological skills, but also
the disturbed marital relationship. As the latter improved, the impairment in his neuropsychological skills was less evident.

It would appear that rehabilitation with the brain-injured, to
be effective, may involve certain standard cognitive retraining
methods, but also an individualized program worked out for each patient on the basis of pre-morbid strengths and weaknesses, as well
as the specific nature of the deficits, preferred learning mode,
methods of rewards and behavioral self-control, and the patient's
personality reaction to the damage (Brinkman, 1979). This is a
costly process, not only financially, but in the dedication and per-
severance of the therapist. Gains are likely to be modest for long
periods of time, but when adaptive behaviors are reestablished, the
therapist's rewards could be tremendous.

Hemispheric Asymmetries

There is little doubt that the 70's will be known as the decade
of hemispheric asymmetries. With the publication in the mid-60s by
Sperry (1968) of the startling evidence for differential hemispheric
functioning in the callosal sectioned patients, journal research in
this area exploded. By mid 1970, we had books published on hemispheric functioning; that is, Gazzaniga's The Bisected Brain (1970);
Dimond's (1972) The Double Brain; Dimond and Beaumont's (1974)
Hemisphere Function in the Human Brain; Harnad et al.'s (1976) Lateralization in the Nervous System; Gazzaniga and LeDoux's (1978)
The Integrated Brain; and, Kinsbourne's (1978) Asymmetrical Function
of the Brain; and an influential section on hemisphere specialization
and interaction appeared in the prestigious Schmitt and Worden's
(1974) The Neurosciences Third Study Program.

By the mid 70's the sequential, analytic, linguistic functions
of the left hemipshere and the holistic, global, synthetic, percept-
ual-spatial skills of the right hemisphere were common knowledge.
Hemispheric asymmetries became the new phrenology (Parsons, 1977),
capable of explaining some of the great mysteries of the nature of
man: the fount of artistic and musical abilities was located in the
right hemisphere; psychodynamicists identified Freud's primary proc-
cess in the right and secondary process in the left hemisphere
(Galin, 1974); humanistic and growth psychologists found that consciousness of sensory qualities and appreciation of sensory input
seemed appropriately located in the primordial Rousseauian right
hemisphere, while the digital, logical, pedantic left hemisphere

exerted a despotic control; a control which could be removed by med-
itation, drugs, alpha training or self-hypnosis; psychopathologists
proposed schizophrenia as left hemisphere and depression as right
hemisphere disorders; theologians found a biological basis for the
ineffable in the proposition that religious experience and spiritual
mysticism emanates from right hemisphere functions; educators seized
the opportunity to emphasize that both hemispheres of the brain had
to be utilized in the educative process and that interhemispheric
difficulties might be responsible from some learning problems; the
origin of consciousness itself was provocatively and brilliantly
postulated by Julian Jaynes (1976) to lie in the breakdown of the
bicameral mind, or stated positively, in the integration of the psychological functions of the two hemispheres.

This professional and increasing secular exploration of the
hemispheres has resulted in an astonishing variety of findings.
Recently, a press release written by a psychologist for a local
newspaper contained a neuropsychological explanation for lateralized
tobacco chewing by baseball players. In a survey conducted with 13
major league teams, the following results were obtained: "Right-
handed ball-players are nearly twice as likely to chew on the left
side as on the right side... left-handers are a troublesome group,
however,.... They are equally likely to chew on the left as on the
right... a respectable sampling of players are undecided...." One
switch hitter chews on the same side as he is hitting from at the
time. The author of the article went on to place the findings in a
neuropsychological context as studies on dominance and laterality.

There is no question that the work on hemispheric asymmetries
has been and will be of great importance in neuropsychology. However, as in the case of many discoveries in science, I believe we
have witnessed the gold rush; the mother lode has been mined and
now two movements are detectable. First, to continue in the analogy,
prospectors are ranging far afield in the hopes of uncovering new
strikes and often find fool's gold or nothing of consequence. Secondly, the remaining ore in the lode can now only be profitably ex-
tracted by intensive and skilled mining operations. In other words,
we are now settling into the period where careful studies must be
done which explicate the hemispheric functions in great detail.

There are three aspects of studies in hemispheric functioning
which I think will dominate much of the work in the near future.
First, the search will continue for a task which gives rise to consistent, across-laboratories repeatable evidence for right hemisphere superiority in normal subjects. Two years ago we surveyed
the literature to locate such a task and decided that Kimura's
(1969) visual dot-location task was the best candidate. This test
involves presentation of a black dot on a white background for a
brief exposure, a post-stimulus mask and then a selection of dot
location from a card with approximately 50 dots on it. We duplicated

her conditions as closely as possible and found to our surprise that
rather than right hemisphere superiority, we actually had a significant overall left hemisphere superiortiy. Further, we found evidence
for an alternation effect in which in early trials the right hemisphere would perform better but in later trials the left hemisphere
would do so. These results are depicted in Figure 1.

Mean number of correct dot locations for 24 trials (12 to each
visual field) is the dependent variable. Set 1 and Set 2 (24 stimulus cards each) were counterbalanced. The whole procedure was repeated three times (tests). As seen in the figure, the left visual
field was better than the right on the first 24 trials of Test I and
II, but reversed on the second 24 trials; by Test III, consistent
right visual field superiority was seen. Not only do these data
raise questions about any unqualified assertion of right hemispheric
superiority on this visual-spatial task independent of variables
such as number of presentations, but also raise the question of shift
of hemispheric attentiveness or strategy over time. A recent report
in Science (Klein & Armitage, 1978) describes 90 to 100 minute oscillations in performance on verbal matching (left hemisphere) and
spatial matching (right hemisphere) tasks over an 8-hour period.
These oscillations were 180° out of phase; that is, when verbal
matching scores were high, spatial scores were relatively low and

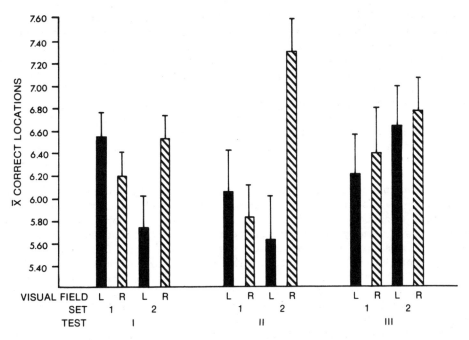

Fig. 1

vice-versa. If these results are replicated, there are clearcut
implications for all studies of hemispheric functioning. To return
to my introductory statement and to paraphrase an old saying, "What
this country needs is a good (reliable) right hemisphere task."

The second focus of hemispheric research will be on the development of asymmetries. Are the hemispheric asymmetries genetically
determined and present at birth, or are they a product of experience;
that is, can hemispheric superiority for a given task be shifted?
There is growing evidence to suggest that hemispheric differences in
response to verbal and nonverbal stimuli exist as early as the first
several weeks in life (Gardiner & Walter, 1977). Such differences
may continue unchanged as growth proceeds. Cioffi and Kandel (1979)
gave children from 7 through 12 a tactual recognition task. For
shapes, the left hand was better; for words the right hand was better.
The differences were similar over the range of ages tested. These
findings plus many others suggest that hemispheric asymmetries are
present at or soon after birth and are maintained throughout development and maturity.

On the other hand, there are reports such as those of Bever and
Chiarello (1974) in which it is suggested that experience can result
in a shift of apparent dominance. In their experiment, musically
experienced subjects performed a musical task (recognition of simple
melodies) better with their right ear (left hemisphere), while musically naive subjects performed better with their left ear (right
hemisphere). Bever and Chiarello (1974) concluded that it was the
kind of processing applied to a musical stimulus which determines
which hemisphere is dominant and that musical experience led to a
shift from right to left hemisphere strategy. If this conclusion
were valid, the potential for education and remediation would be
tremendous. However, the evidence for genetic determination of musical ability is quite strong and a more parsimonious explanation of
the Bever and Chiarello results is possible. Assuming that high aptitude would result in greater musical experience, and that aptitude
is related to the left hemisphere's superiority, then the experience
of the subjects would be a concomitant, not a causal, factor.

We administered two tests of musical ability monaurally to subjects who were selected on the basis of aptitude and experience
(Parsons, Gaede, & Bertera, 1979). Test 1 was a chord analysis test;
Test 2 was a memory for sequence test. Each S performed both tests
with each ear in a predetermined order. There were 59 Ss, approximately equal males and females. The results are depicted in Figure
1 in the left-hand figure. Test 1 and Test 2 differed significantly
on the left ear minus right ear measure (F = 7.18, p <.01), Test 1
showing a right hemisphere superiortiy; Test 2 a left hemisphere
superiority. The interaction of aptitude and the ear difference
measure just missed significance (F = 3.85, p < .07), but the effect
was clearly in the low aptitude subjects; that is, high aptitude sub-

jects performed each test equally well in either ear, whereas low aptitude Ss appeared to do better with the hemisphere whose strategy was more appropriate for the task. In contrast to aptitude, experience had not significant effect on the ear difference score. We suggest that aptitude, presumably genetically determined, rather than experience, is the important determinant of hemispheric asymmetry.

The third area of hemispheric research is that of gender differences. There is a growing body of literature suggesting differences between males and females in perceptual-cognitive functioning (Mac-

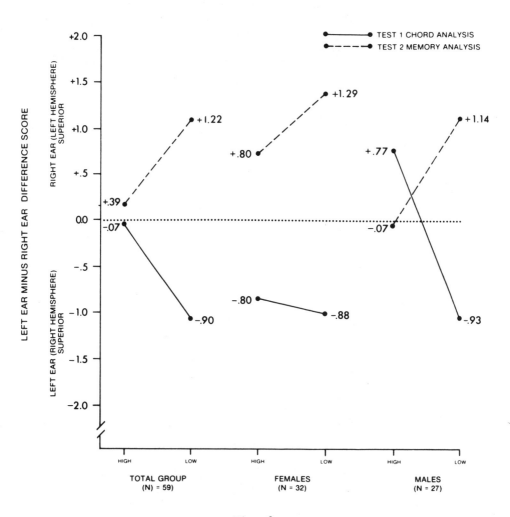

Fig. 2

coby & Jacklin, 1974). Males typically do better on tasks involving
visual-spatial skills, thought to be more salient in the right hemisphere, while females have greater verbal skills; processes salient
in the left hemisphere. Secondly, males and females may differ in
degree of functional asymmetry of the brain. Most evidence suggests
that males exhibit stronger lateralization than females, particularly
for right hemisphere dependent activities (McGlone, 1978; Witelson,
1976).

     In our experiment with musical ability, we found sex differences.
As seen on the right side of Figure 1, males had a significant inter-
action between aptitude and ear difference score ($\underline{F}$ = 4.09, $\underline{p}$ <.05),
but non-significant overall differences on tests. Does this mean a
greater genetic contribution to the hemispheric asymmetries on musical tasks in males than females? Females had a significant differ-
ence on tests ($\underline{F}$ = 5.16, $\underline{p}$ <.05), but no interaction of aptitude and
tests. Do these results mean greater hemispheric lateralization in
females than males? If so, the results are at variance with the conclusions summarized earlier. Obviously, there is much experimentation
lying ahead to unravel these complexities.

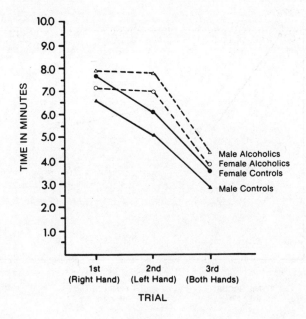

Fig. 3

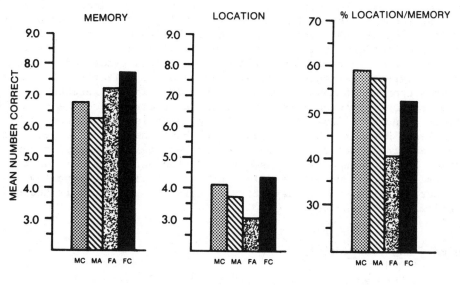

Fig. 4

In another study, we have explored the differential effects of chronic alcoholism on tactual-spatial performance by males and females. The Tactual-Performance Test (TPT) (Time) from the HRB has consistently discriminated alcoholics from non-alcoholics (Parsons & Farr, 1981). We tested the hypothesis that (1) alcoholism has a relatively greater effect on functions of the right hemisphere than the left, and (2) that this effect would be more pronounced in males than females (Fabian, Jenkins, & Parsons, 1981). The TPT was administered in standard fashion (right hand, left hand, and both hands). The results for TPT-Time are depicted in Figure 3. Alcoholics performed significantly more poorly than controls (F = 7.62, p < .01); the differences between right hand performances did not achieve significance, while those of the left hand were markedly different (F = 15.53, p < .001); finally, there was a significant Sex x Alcoholism interaction (F = 4.10, p < .05), indicating that the effect of alcoholism on TPT was not the same for males and females. As seen in Figure 3, control males were far superior to alcoholic males (F = 15.89, p < .001), but the performance of female alcoholics and controls were not different.

On the Memory for Shapes measure, women remembered more shapes, as can be seen in Figure 4, than men (F = 9.59, p < .01), but alcoholism had no main effect. On the Location measure, also depicted in Figure 4, there was a main effect of alcoholism (F = 3.86, p <.05), but not of sex. However, females overall had significantly poorer percent location scores than males (F = 5.12, p <.05). Many of our findings support the contention that alcoholism has a relatively greater effect on right hemisphere functioning than on the left. However, what can be said about the hypothesized gender differences; that is, greater effects in males than females? Clearly, the answer depends upon which measure is used. For TPT-Time differences in level of performance between male alcoholics and their controls and the lack of differences in females, argues for greater lateralization effects in males. However, the left hand-right hand analysis revealed a similar pattern in males and females. Further, females actually performed better than males on memory, but then performed more poorly on percent location, with female alcoholics having the lowest scores! In short, in hemispheric asymmetry research, there are multitudinous problems to be resolved.

Summary and Prospects

The "new emergent speciality" of clinical neuropsychology for which I optimistically predicted a healthy growth in 1970, has been realized and far surpassed my expectations. Clinical neuropsychological assessment laboratories and services have become part and parcel of better health care delivery organizations; to a large extent this has been due to workers using the Halstead-Reitan Battery and from the development of special techniques for children and the elderly. The next decade will see these techniques tested for efficacy under a variety of conditions with many different populations. There will be an increasing number of neuropsychology laboratories established. With this expansion will come professional problems, such as the greater demand for neuropsychologists to testify in court as regards their findings in patients with possible or known brain damage who are involved in litigation. This development has implications for the training of neuropsychologists of the future.

Also, during the next decade there will be a major commitment of professional effort to rehabilitation and cognitive-perceptual retraining. Progress here is likely to be slow and demanding with no easy solutions or short cuts. Scientifically based programs which are individualized, flexible, and behavioral but holistically oriented are likely to be most effective in treatment. Case studies with specific details as to retraining methods and strategies will be helpful during this period; perhaps a greater leniency of Journal editors in this regard would facilitate progress.

Research on hemispheric asymmetries, the most popular neuropsychological research on the last decade, will continue with the limitations and advantages gradually delineated by the systematic, orderly process which constitutes so much of science. In my opinion, the problems which will receive the most attention are: 1) the development of a reliable, inter-laboratory repeatable right hemisphere task; 2) the developmental course and modifiability of hemispheric asymmetries; and, 3) gender effects in hemispheric functioning. Of course, there are many other research areas not covered in this review which will receive attention and provide impetus for new directions.

The growth and development of clinical neuropsychology rests on a firm foundation. At the interface between the psychological and biological sciences, neuropsychology is in a position on the one hand to contribute to the applied problems of the clinic and, on the other hand, to contribute to the explication of what has been termed "the last frontier," the human brain and mind.

REFERENCES

Aaron, P.G. A neuropsychological key approach to diagnosis and re-mediation of learning disabilities. Journal of Clinical Psychology, 1979, 35, 326-335.

Ben-Yishay, Y. Working approaches to remediation of cognitive deficits in brain-damaged. Supplements to 6th and 7th Annual Workshops for Rehabilitation Professionals, June, 1978, May, 1979. Institute of Rehabilitation Medicine, New York University Medical Center, Department of Behavioral Sciences.

Bever, T.G. & Chiarello, R.J. Cerebral dominance in musicians and non-musicians. Science, 1974, 185, 537-539.

Boll, T.J. Diagnosing brain impairment. In B. Wolman, Clinical diagnosis of mental disorders. New York: Plenum Press, 1978.

Brinkman, S.D. Rehabilitation of the neurologically impaired patient: The contributions of the neuropsychologist. Clinical Neuropsychology, 1979, 1, 39-44.

Christensen, A.L. Luria's neuropsychological investigation. New York: Spectrum, 1975a.

Christensen, A.L. Luria's neuropsychological investigation: Manual. New York: Spectrum, 1975b.

Cioffi, J., & Kandel, G.L. Laterality of stereognostic accuracy of children for words, shapes and bigrams. Science, 1979, 204, 1431-1434.

Dimond, S.J. The double brain. London: Churchill Livingstone, 1972.

Dimond, S.J., & Beaumont, J. (Eds.) Hemisphere function in the human brain. New York: John Wiley & Sons, 1974.

Fabian, M.S., Jenkins, R.L., & Parsons, O.A. Gender, alcoholism and neuropsychological functioning. Journal of Consulting and Clinical Psychology, 1981, 41, 139-141.

Galin, D. Implications for psychiatry of left and righ cerebral specialization. Archives of General Psychiatry, 1974, 31, 572-583.

Gardiner, M.D., & Walter, D.O. Evidence of hemispheric specializa-
    tion from infant EEG. In S. Harnad et al. (Eds.), Lateraliza-
    tion in the nervous system. New York: Academic Press, 1977.

Gazzaniga, M.D., & LeDoux, J.E. The integrated mind. New York:
    Plenum Press, 1978.

Gazzaniga, M.S. The bisected brain. New York: Appleton-Century-
    Crofts, 1970.

Glasgow, R.E., Zeiss, R.A., Barrera, M., & Lewinsohn, P.M. Case
    studies on remediating memory deficits in brain damaged indi-
    viduals. Journal of Clinical Psychology, 1977, 33, 1049-1054.

Golden, C.J. Validity of the Halstead Reitan Neuropsychological
    Battery in a mixed psychiatric and brain-injured population.
    Journal of Consulting and Clinical Psychology, 1977, 45, 1043-
    1051.

Golden, C.J. Diagnosis and rehabilitation in clinical neuropsy-
    chology. Springfield, Ill: Charles E. Thomas, 1978.

Golden, C.J., Hammeke, T.A., & Purisch, A.D. Diagnostic validity
    of a standardized neuropsychological battery derived from Luria's
    Neuropsychological Tests. Journal of Consulting and Clinical
    Psychology, 1978, 46, 1258-1265.

Golden, C. Standardized Luria's Neuropsychological evaluation: Fur-
    ther clinical and experimental results. Symposium at the 87th
    Annual Meeting of the American Psychological Association, New
    York City, September, 1979.

Golden, C.J. A standardized version of Luria's neuropsychological
    tests. In S. Filskov, & T. Boll, Handbook of clinical neuro-
    psychology. New York: John Wiley & Sons, 1981.

Goldstein, G. Methodological and theoretical issues in neuropsych-
    ological assessment. Journal of Behavioral Assessment, 1979,
    1, 23-41.

Goldstein, K. After-effects of brain-injury in war. New York:
    Grune & Stratton, 1942.

Hécaen, H., & Albert, M.L. Human neuropsychology. New York: John
    Wiley & Sons, 1978.

Halstead, W.C. Brain and intelligence. Chicago: University of
    Chicago Press, 1947.

Harnad, S., Doty, R.W., Goldstein, L., Jaynes, J., & Krauthamer, G.
    Lateralization in the nervous system. New York: Academic Press,
    1976.

Heaton, R.K., Smith, H.A., Lehman, R.A., & Vogt, A.T. The prospects
    for faking believeable deficits on neuropsychological testing.
    Journal of Consulting and Clinical Psychology, 1978, 46, 892-900.

Heilman, K.M., & Valenstein, E. Clinical neuropsychology. New York:
    Oxford University Press, 1979.

Horton, A.M., Jr. Behavioral neuropsychology: Rationale and research.
    Clinical Neuropsychology, 1979, 1, 20-24.

Jaynes, J. The origin of consciousness in the breakdown of the bi-
    cameral mind. Boston: Houghton-Mifflin Co., 1976.

Kane, R.L., Moses, J., & Sweet, J. Comparison of the Luria Neuro-
    psychological Battery and the Halstead Reitan. Paper presented

in Golden, Colorado. Standardized Luria neuropsychological evaluation: Further clinical and experimental results. Symposium at the 87th Annual Meeting of the American Psychological Association, New York City, September, 1979.

Kaszniak, A.W., Kelly, M., & Schneider, A. Reliability and validity of a neuropsychological screening battery for older adults. Paper presented at the 31st Annual Scientific Meeting of the Gerontological Society, November, 1978, Dallas, Texas.

Kimura, D. Spatial localization in left and right visual fields. Canadian Journal of Psychology, 1969, 23, 445-458.

Kinsbourne, M. Asymmetrical function of the brain. New York: Cambridge University Press, 1978.

Klein, R., & Armitage, R. Rhythms in human performance: 1½ hour oscillations in cognitive style. Science, 1978, 204, 1326-1327.

Lewinsohn, P.M., Danaher, B., & Kikel, S. Visual imagery as a mnemonic aid for brain-injured persons. Journal of Consulting and Clinical Psychology, 1977, 45, 717-723.

Lewinsohn, P.M., Glasgow, R.E., Barrera, M., Danaher, B.G., Alperson, J., McCarty, D.L., Sullivan, J.M., Zeiss, R.A., Nyland, J., & Rodrigues, M.R.P. Assessment and treatment of patients with memory deficits: Initial studies. JSAS Catalogue of Selected Documents in Psychology, 1977, 7, 79.

Lezak, M.D. Neuropsychological assessment. New York: Oxford University Press, 1976.

Luria, A.R. Higher cortical functions in man. New York: Basic Books, 1966.

Luria, A.R., & Majovski, L.V. Basic approaches used in American and Soviet clinical neuropsychology. American Psychologist, 1977, 32, 959-968.

Luria, A.R., Naydin, V.L., Tsvetkova, L.S., & Vinarskaya. Restoration of higher cortical function following local brain damage. In P. J. Vinken, & G.W. Bruyn (Eds.), Handbook of clinical neurology 3. Disorders of higher nervous activity. New York: American Elsevier Publishing Co., 1969.

McGlone, J. Sex differences in functional brain asymmetry. Cortex, 1978, 14, 122-128.

Maccoby, E.E., & Jacklin, C.N. The psychology of sex differences. Stanford, CA: Stanford University Press, 1974.

Parsons, O.A. Clinical neuropsychology. In C.D. Spielberger (Ed.), Current topics in clinical and community psychology, Vol. 2. New York: Academic Press, 1970.

Parsons, O.A. Human neuropsychology: The new phrenology. Journal of Operational Psychiatry, 1977, 8, 47-56.

Parsons, O.A. Clinical neuropsychology: Past, present, and future. Talk given at Emery John Brady Hospital, Colorado Springs, Colorado, February, 1978.

Parsons, O.A., & Farr, S.P. Neuropsychology of alcohol and drug use. In S. Filskov & T. Boll (Eds.), Handbook of clinical neuropsychology. New York: John Wiley & Sons, 1981.

Parsons, O.A., Gaede, S.E., & Bertera, J.H. Effects of gender, aptitude and experience on hemispheric asymmetries in music perception. Biological Psychology Bulletin, 1979, 5, 149-160.

Parsons, O.A., & Prigatano, G.P. Methodological considerations in clinical neuropsychological research. Journal of Consulting and Clinical Psychology, 1978, 46, 608-619.

Prigatano, G.P. Neuropsychological recovery patterns of a young head injury patient with aphasia. Paper presented at the European Conference of the International Neuropsychology Society, Oxford, England, August, 1977.

Purisch, D., Golden, C.J., & Hammeke, T.A. Discrimination of schizophrenic and brain-injured patients by a standardized version of Luria's Neuropsychological Tests. Journal of Consulting and Clinical Psychology, 1978, 46, 1266-1273.

Reitan, R.M., & Davison, L.A. (Eds.) Clinical neuropsychology: Current status and applications. New York: John Wiley & Sons, 1974.

Russell, E., Neuringer, C., & Goldstein, G. Assessment of brain damage: A neuropsychological key approach. New York: John Wiley & Sons, 1970.

Schmitt, F.O., & Worden, F.G. (Eds.) The neurosciences, third study program. Cambridge: Massachusetts Institute of Technology Press, 1974.

Selz, M., & Reitan, R. Rules for neuropsychological diagnosis: Classification of brain functions in older children. Journal of Consulting and Clinical Psychology, 1979, 47. 258-264.

Small, L. Neuropsychodiagnosis in psychotherapy. New York: Brunner/ Mazel, 1973.

Sollee, N. Clinical neuropsychology services in a pediatric hospital. Symposium presented at the 87th Annual Meeting of the American Psychological Association, New York City, September, 1979.

Sperry, R.W. Hemispheric deconnection and unity in conscious awareness. American Psychologist, 1968, 23, 723-733.

Witelson, S. Sex and the single hemisphere: Specialization of the right hemisphere for spatial processing. Science, 1976, 193, 425-427.

SPONTANEOUS RECOVERY AND EFFICACY OF THERAPY IN APHASIA

Nancy Helm-Estabrooks and Audrey L. Holland

Veterans Administration Medical Center, Boston, and
The University of Pittsburgh, Pittsburgh

To the aphasiologist who has been involved in treatment and has witnessed the return of some significant amount of language in her aphasic patient, possibly the five most frustrating words in the English language are "He'd have gotten better anyway." Often uttered by physicians who are doubtful about the efficacy of treatment, they further represent an unwarranted optimism regarding the effects of spontaneous recovery. The underlying assumption of this paper is that spontaneous recovery and treatment are partners in effecting the best possible recovery from aphasia. The purposes are to describe what is known concerning spontaneous recovery from aphasia and to discuss the evidence attesting to the efficacy of treatment. In this way, the interactive nature of the two processes, one naturally-occurring and the other representing human manipulation, can each be better understood.

Spontaneous Recovery

Immediately following a stroke or other aphasia-producing event, the aphasic person's language disorder is at its worst. Both the severity of the event and the extent of brain damage produced contribute to this temporarily bleak picture. Within a few days, however, the natural recovery process begins. Spontaneous recovery is influenced by a number of factors, including age, extent and location of the brain damage, general condition of the patient, and to some degree, the quality of care a patient receives. In the main, however, spontaneous recovery is an inevitable physiological repair process, the attempt of the brain to resume its normal function.

Rubens (1977) describes the physical events of the spontaneous

41

recovery process first by summarizing the changes that occur in the brain immediately following a stroke or other brain damage. These changes are akin to a "shut down" process:

1. The brain swells; edema sets in.
2. Blood flow to both hemispheres is reduced.
3. Disproportionately large amounts of inhibitory neurotrans-
    mitters (catecholamines) are released.
4. Diaschisis begins. That is, generalized effects of disrup-
    tion to a part of the previously patent brain begin to make
    themselves felt. Temporary suspension of functions occurs
    in parts of the brain far removed from the site of trouble.

Rubens (1977) argues that spontaneous recovery is the reversal of these "holding" processes. Over time, parts of the brain undam-aged by the cerebral episode return to normal functioning. Specifi-cally:

1. Edema lessens.
2. Blood flow is normalized, certainly to the undamaged hemis-
    phere.
3. Catecholamine levels return to normal.
4. Normal function in undamaged brain areas is resumed. That
    is, the effects of diaschisis are minimized.

In short, the physiological events of spontaneous recovery are related to the ability of the undamaged remainder of the brain to approximate normal functioning.

Spontaneous recovery continues for 3-6 months or longer, and with it the expectation of improvement of the aphasic condition. The process is most rapid relatively soon after the damaged brain has become stabilized, and as time progresses the rate of change shows a negatively accelerating course. The pattern of spontaneous recovery during this period is likely to be related to the type of insult that produced the aphasia in the first place. For example, ischemic stroke patients show a relatively smooth negative acceler-ation course; hemorrhagic stroke patients often begin the spontaneous recovery process somewhat later and improve more rapidly once the process is started; head-trauma patients have been noted by Porch (1971) to show abrupt changes, followed by brief periods of no im-provement, then abrupt changes again, and so on.

The spontaneous changes during this period occur not only in language abilities, but in most of the cognitive, motor and sensory disabilities that might accompany aphasia as well. It is of inter-est, then, that most of the studies of spontaneous recovery of func-tion have involved clearly aphasic patients, and have centered upon the recovery of language abilities. One reason for this dispropor-tionate emphasis on the aphasic symptomatology is probably due to interest in the efficacy of treatment of aphasia. It is clear that good spontaneous recovery data are crucial to adequate assessment of the effects of treatment. Meier (1974) summarizes the relationship as follows:

> Naturally occuring lesions in patients with acute cerebral infarctions due to cerebrovascular disease may provide more appropriate baseline data for monitoring the longitudinal course of recovery, particularly if the baseline can be established early in the recovery period, before spontaneous changes have arisen... (Such assessment strategies)... might help delineate the boundary conditions within which behavior modification and rehabilitation procedures can be introduced.

Although Meier was speaking generally about restitution of cortical function, the applicability of his statements specifically to aphasia is obvious.

A number of retrospective studies (Vignolo, 1964; Keenan & Brassell, 1974; Brust, Shafer, Rechter, & Braun, 1976; Kertesz & McCabe, 1977; Lomas & Kertesz, 1978; Porch, Collins, Wertz, & Fridan, 1980), have examined recovery patterns of adults with aphasia. As a group, these studies show that auditory comprehension is most likely to recover. For example, even though the Porch et al. (1980) study, using the Porch Index of Communicative Ability (PICA) (1971), as the evaluation instrument, showed gestural subtest scores to be the best predictor of outcome, the authors attributed the gestural changes to increased ability to "listen." As a group, these retrospective studies also show that maximal gains occur in the first three months post-ictus.

Prospective studies, that is, studies which identify aphasia patients early and follow their progress for some time, have also been carried out (Culton, 1969; Kenin & Swisher, 1972; Ludlow, 1977; Levita, 1978; Demeurisse et al., 1980). The prospective studies usually involve smaller samples than do retrospective studies, but show general agreement with them in suggesting that maximal improvement occurs in the first three months. However, the work of Sarno and Levita (1971) and Demeurisse et al. (1980), the two studies which followed patients from the earliest time post onset, fail to show the superiority in auditory comprehension gain over speech production gain.

With the exceptions noted below, the majority of the prospective and retrospective studies have common features which open them to criticism and limit their generality. First, most used a variety of aphasia tests that were standardized on chronic, as opposed to acutely, aphasic patients. The exceptions are Demeurisse et al.

(1980), and Culton (1969), who used tests designed especially for their studies (and for which they presented no reliability data). The use of instruments designed for the chronically aphasic raises questions regarding generalizing data obtained from them to the newly-brain damaged. That is, the instruments themselves may affect the outcomes of the studies. For example, the Lomas and Kertesz (1978) study found that both initially fluent and non-fluent patients showed gains in auditory comprehension regardless of the initial level of comprehension. In that study, some patients were tested with an hour-long formal test only one day post-stroke, using a test with reliability calculated, naturally enough, on only chronic patients. Confusion, disorientation, and even simple illness, all potentially affect comprehension and can confound formal measures of that ability.

A second critical feature is that, with the exception of Sarno and Levita (1971, 1979), (and a few questionable patients like the Lomas and Kertesz (1978) patient just described), all of the studies involved patients late enough in the recovery process already to have been classified as aphasic. This means that there is virtually no baseline spontaneous recovery data on patients who have cognitive or other deficits as a result of right-hemispheric damage, or whose aphasia quickly resolves.

Mohr's (1973) study of three patients is a clear exception to these criticisms. Mohr began studying these patients immediately post-stroke, at regular intervals during hospitalization, and less frequently thereafter. Using simple nonstandardized bedside tests he reported these patients' as having unique, quick-resolving non-fluent aphasias. He eventually correlated the initial deficits and their resolutions to the patients' neuropathology at autopsy. The study stands as a useful model of the type of research that is needed to fully understand the general natural outcomes in aphasia, as well as other cognitive deficits following brain damage.

The literature suggests that, with or without intervention, the severity of aphasia lessens in the first three months post onset and auditory comprehension change is most likely to occur spontaneously through that period. Beyond that, little is clearly known. Limitations exist on what is known concerning the outcomes of spontaneous recovery. We suggest it is an area worthy of more thorough investigation.

Spontaneous Recovery and Evolution of Aphasic Symptomatology

There are several studies in which aphasic patients are identified early, and are followed for some time, usually at least a year post-onset. Typically in such studies, patients are receiving treatment; making it virtually impossible to distinguish the effects of spontaneous recovery itself from the effects of treatment. Nonetheless, these studies offer some intriguing insights into the changing nature of aphasia over time.

Reinvang and Engvik (1980), studied 33 patients and found that for 22 of them the presenting aphasic classification was retained 3-6 months post-onset, although there was a reduction in severity. In contrast, Kertesz and McCabe (1977), studied 93 patients for one year post-onset; some unspecified number of the patients received treatment, some did not. Of these 93, 22 recovered completely. Of the remaining 71, only 27 retained their initial aphasia classification. Of particular interest is the fact that the predominant evolution was to anomic aphasia, which Kertesz and McCabe (1977) described as being "a common end state in evolution, in addition to being a common aphasic syndrome de novo." They noted this evolution from previously Wernicke, transcortical, Broca, conduction and global patients. Wertz, Kitselman, and Deal (1981), perhaps more appropriately describing changes in type of aphasia as "migrations" rather than "evolutions," have produced strikingly similar findings in a large group of treated aphasic patients.

A fascinating related finding has recently been reported by Sarno and Levita (1979), who followed carefully-selected global aphasic patients for a year post-onset. They reported that their patients greatest gains began at six months post-onset, and continued through the end of the year of study. This study indicated that for the most seriously impaired aphasic patients not only spontaneous recovery, but also the effects of treatment, may not begin to surface until, in comparison to other aphasic patients, the period of maximal gain may reasonably be assumed to have already been completed.

The practical implications of these studies for the clinical aphasiologist is that, regardless of when the patient was evaluated (at least in the first year post-onset), the clinician must be aware of the potential for change in severity and form of aphasia. There is an overall trend toward lessening of severity, as well as toward less devastating forms of aphasia. Periodic reassessment is crucial. Changes in symptomatology may necessitate a change in therapeutic strategy, geared to the new pattern of language performance.

For those who are committed to the value of treatment, the issue of when to begin treatment is also related to spontaneous recovery. On one hand, it can be logically argued that maximally beneficial treatment should begin early; thereby capitalizing upon spontaneous gains. On the other hand, waiting for direct intervention, until the condition has stabilized, can potentially be more efficient; particularly if, during that period, supportive counseling is provided. Moreover, as shown in Sarno and Levita's (1979) study of global patients, the effects of early intervention were not reflected in gains

until six months or more had elapsed. While most clinical aphasiologists have a strong commitment to the belief that the optimal time
for intervention is early in the recovery process, no hard data have
been generated in support of this belief.

If one wishes to conduct research on the efficacy of treatment,
it is best to initiate the treatment after the period of greatest
spontaneous recovery has elapsed. In this way, improvement can be
attributed to the therapy -- not simply to natural change. For individual aphasic patients, the issue of when to initiate treatment
is less clear, although both family and patients should be counseled
and supported as soon as possible after the onset of aphasia.

Efficacy of Treatment

It has been argued that some degree of spontaneous recovery is
a natural consequence of having become aphasic in the first place.
Unfortunately, many aphasic patients fail to improve spontaneously
to a level of functional communication or to a level which allows
them to resume pre-aphasia vocational, social and self-care activities. The issue then becomes one of rehabilitation.

The first report of aphasia rehabilitation was made by Trosseau
in 1864 (Riese, 1947), of an amnesic aphasic patient who re-educated
her own speech. She began by repeating the speech of others which
revived the memory of spoken words. Later she recorded words produced by herself and others in a notebook. The first detailed description of aphasia therapy approaches appeared in 1904. The author
was Charles Mills, an American physician. Mills (1904) apparently
became interested in aphasia rehabilitation when a patient who came
to him two years post-onset of aphasia made "remarkable advances"
in several months' time through "the most persistent efforts to re-
educate his stricken brain." When he reported this and other cases
to the 55th annual session of the American Medical Association, a
Dr. C.W. Burr remarked that "it is very hard for us to say how much
of the improvement is due to education and how much is due to the
natural course of events" (Mills, 1904). This same skepticism regarding the efficacy of aphasia therapy continues to persist in the
medical community some 75 years later. Pryse-Phillips (1980), has
stated: "The place of speech therapy in rehabilitation (of hemiplegic
patients) is in dispute." In 1979, however, the neurologist Frank
Benson concluded his review of a large aphasia treatment study by
stating "the findings... strongly suggest that therapy does affect
recovery from aphasia."

One way of resolving the dispute regarding aphasia rehabilitation
is to examine the evidence which suggests, or better yet proves, that
aphasia therapy can effect a greater degree or better quality of improvement than can be expected through natural recovery alone. There

are several ways of obtaining this evidence. Two of those ways will
be discussed briefly here:

> 1. Group studies of treated and untreated patients.
> 2. Case studies of untreated then treated patients.

Group Studies of Aphasia Rehabilitation

Group studies of aphasia rehabilitation compare well-matched
samples of patients who are first identified and classified as aphasic, and then are randomly placed either in a treatment group or are
left totally untreated. Many health care agencies, however, believe
that treatment is better than no treatment. To them, denial of treatment is unethical; therefore, the ideal study is difficult to carry
out. Nonetheless, natural events often provide the opportunity for
this study design.

The first opportunity to compare untreated and treated patients
occurred during World War II in the United States. Due to either
physician skepticism or to a bureaucratic error, a group of aphasic
veterans was not transferred to the newly developed aphasia unit at
an army hospital (Eisenson, 1949). When "discovered" some 8 months
later, Eisenson found that their language recovery compared unfavor-
ably with the patients who had been receiving treatment. In addition, a sense of discouragement and even "psychological problems"
seemed to exist within the untreated group. Of course, Eisenson did
not have pre-test scores for this group, so his serendipitous study
can qualify only as an interesting observation.

Naturally occurring evidence has also allowed for an ongoing
Italian study of treated and untreated groups of aphasic patients
(Basso, Faglioni, & Vignolo, 1975; Basso, Capitani, & Vignolo, 1979).
The untreated group comprised patients who were evaluated formally
after onset of aphasia, but because of what were primarily geographic
reasons were unable to travel to rehabilitation centers for language
therapy. The 1975 study reported on 94 treated and 94 untreated
patients who were rated on a 4-point recovery scale. When retested,
the untreated group failed to show recovery patterns equal to those
of the treated group.

By 1979, 162 treated patients and 119 untreated controls had
been studied. The times post-onset for initial testing was 0-2
months for 137 cases, 2-6 months for 86 cases, and more than 6 months
for 58 cases. All patients were retested at least 6 months later.
The group who had received a minimum of 3 treatment sessions per week
during that period made greater gains in speaking, listening, writing
and reading than the untreated group did.

In a serendipitous study which occurred within the context of test development, Holland (1980) discovered that chronically aphasic patients who were continued in therapy showed significantly improved second-testing scores on a test of functional communication (Communicative Abilities in Daily Living Measure, 1980). A group who had been discontinued from therapy failed to show improvement.

Perhaps the only study to report that treated and untreated patients could not be differentiated on the basis of changes in test scores over time was carried out by Levita (1979). Using the Functional Communication Profile (Sarno, 1969), Levita compared 17 patients treated at a rehabilitation institute with 18 patients consequently admitted to a general hospital. The treated group was considered "chronic," while the untreated group was apparently acute. In view of issues previously discussed, the problems in comparing these two populations become obvious.

The ethical issue of purposefully denying treatment to aphasic patients was addressed in a recent Veterans Administration Study (Wertz et al., 1981). Fifty-eight patients who met strict criteria for inclusion were randomly assigned to one of the two groups. Group A received individualized language therapy. Group B entered a social interaction group. Pre- and post-treatment scores earned on the Porch Index of Communicative Ability (Porch, 1971) were compared for the groups. Both groups showed considerable improvement with Group A showing slightly better gains.

Canter (1971) was speaking of stuttering research when he said that:

> Statistical techniques tell us only about the means of the populations. Individual differences are utilized statistically as error terms. Findings that emerge from studies of differing central tendencies have certain undeniable statistical and conceptual significance, but they have virtually no meaning clinically.

Canter's observation holds true for aphasia research as well as for stuttering. Fortunately, aphasiologists have long recognized the value of good case studies, not only for delineating specific aphasia syndromes, but for testing the effectiveness of aphasia therapy.

Case Studies of Aphasia Rehabilitation

If aphasic patients fail to improve significantly during the period of greatest spontaneous recovery without treatment, but respond positively to treatment at some point after that period, then one has good evidence that the positive change was a result of the

therapy. One such early case was reported by Singer and Low (1933).
These physicians saw a woman who two years after onset of aphasia had
persistent severe hemiplegia and aphasia. Although her comprehension
was good, her verbal output consisted of the stereotype "0-dee-dar."
Using the available "ee" sound as a first step in treatment, Singer
helped her combine "ee" with a blowing sound to produce "bee." This
led to "bar," "bed," "bowl," "book," etc. Within months, the patient
was able to articulate multisyllable words.

By today's standards, Singer and Low's report does not qualify
as a controlled study because they do not provide pre- and post-therapy test data. Instead, the first controlled study of treatment effects was contributed by Weisenburg and McBride (1935). They described a 45-year-old woman with predominantly expressive aphasia
characteristized by marked articulation and word formation problems
with a tendency to omit "less important" words. The patient was
first tested two weeks post-onset. She remained untreated for 7
months, at which time the test was readministered. Although she had
made good improvement in the areas of auditory comprehension, reading and writing, her speaking showed very little improvement. She
was given 6 months of therapy directed at improving articulation and
verbal expression and writing with the left hand (nonpreferred). A
third test showed improvement in speech output, as well as gains in
other areas. A comparison of the earlier no treatment period with
the later treatment period indicated that there had been "far more
improvement during the 6 months of training than during the first 7
months after the attack."

A more severely impaired case is described by Albert, Goodglass,
Helm, Rubens, and Alexander (1981). A 41-year-old aphasic male produced only a few stereotyped phonemes ("dis dis," "kin dis") ten
months post-onset, despite a period of traditional therapy during
the first 3 months. Within two weeks of daily sessions of melodic
intonation therapy introduced in the eleventh month, the patient
spontaneously began to produce meaningful single syllable words.
With approximately 4 months of melodic intonation therapy, he was
communicating through short appropriate sentences as measured by
the Boston Diagnostic Aphasia Examination (Goodglass, & Kaplan,
1972).

Perhaps the most impressive example of improvement with treatment was reported by Basso, Capitani, and Vignolo (1979). These
investigators describe a 49-year-old woman with Broca'a aphasia who
was untreated for eleven years at which time she learned of the rehabilitation unit in Milan. She moved to Milan to enter a course of
treatment. Before treatment, her nonfluent aphasia was characterized
by short, syllabic fragments, marked slowness, long pauses and artic-
ulatory fatigue. Auditory comprehension was fairly good. After 5
sessions of therapy per week for 8 months, her verbal expression,
although still slow with occasional errors, was "flawless in grammar

and meaning." Basso, Capitani, and Vignolo (1979) supply pre- and post-therapy conversation transcripts to support their conclusion that therapy can bring about dramatic improvement even eleven years post-onset of aphasia.

It should be pointed out that all of the cases cited above presented with severe, non-fluent but non-global aphasic syndromes. The patients' auditory comprehension skills far exceeded their verbal expression skills. Our methods for treating this population of aphasic patients are more successful than our methods for treating aphasic syndromes, such as global aphasia and Wernicke's aphasia, which include severe auditory comprehension deficits as part of their symptom complex. There have been some recent advances in treating globally aphasic patients with a highly structured, nonverbal, gestural oriented approach called Visual Action Therapy (Helm-Estabrooks, Fitzpatrick, & Barresi, 1982). At best, however, Visual Action Therapy raises global patients to a level where they can respond to treatment for non-fluent aphasia. This, in turn, may rehabilitate their communication to a more functional level.

Fortunately, for those who are now or who may become aphasic, the field of aphasia rehabilitation is not static. Ongoing exploration of brain-behavior relationships and the communication process is contributing to improved magagement of aphasic patients.

To illustrate this point, the following case is offered. B, a 45-year-old bookkeeper, was admitted to the Boston Veterans Administration Medical Center in January, 1975, with right hemiplegia and non-fluent aphasia. Boston Diagnostic Aphasia Examination one month later showed that his auditory comprehension was moderately well preserved, but his verbal output consisted mainly of the stereotype "see-foos-see-foos." He began a course of melodic intonation therapy (Sparks, Helm, & Albert, 1974), and was discharged with good auditory comprehension and functional production of mainly substantive words. He received no treatment for the next five years. During that time a treatment for agrammatism was developed based upon the research of Gleason and her colleagues (1975). The treatment approach proved successful with one agrammatic patient at three years post-onset of aphasia (Helm-Estabrooks, Fitzpatrick, & Baressi, 1981). B agreed to be readmitted for a trial of what was called the Syntax Stimulation Program for agrammatism. Five years after his initial discharge he produced the following description of the Boston Diagnostic exam cookie theft picture:

> 6/24/80
> "tookie jars-falling down-and-girl-handin some cookie jar-mother's doing dishes-and fall-water-fall-fall."

B then entered a four and a half month course of treatment which trained him to produce eleven sentence types according to a hierarchy of difficulty. Of course, the B.D.A.E. cookie theft picture was not used during this time. Following the syntax stimulation program, he offered the following description:

> 11/30/80
> "The woman is drying the dishes-The boy is reaching tookie jar... give to the girl. The boy-the-tripping. The water flowed-over the floor. The-no-shut faucet off." (Barresi & Helm-Estabrooks, 1981)

This case serves to demonstrate several points regarding aphasia therapy:

1. Evidence obtained from new research in related areas (e.g., neurolinguistic) can provide the basis for new rehabilitation techniques.
2. A rehabilitation approach which proves to be successful for a specific aphasic syndrome, should be effective with other patients displaying that syndrome.
3. If a method is appropriate for a particular aphasic patient, it should effect significant improvement even years after the onset of aphasia.

There is, of course, more to aphasia rehabilitation than applying specific approaches to specific syndromes. Aphasia is a devastating disorder. Aphasia compromises our ability to understand and use spoken language, the very skill which makes us uniquely human. If a patient is not given the opportunity to work through the sense of loss which invariably accompanies the aphasia, then even our best therapies are ineffective. The opportunity to deal with the socio-psychological aspects of aphasia is probably best presented within a group setting. At the Boston Veterans Administration Medical Center, an aphasia discussion group has been thriving for over 4 years (Blair, Walsh, & Cerny, 1979). Originally started by a social worker, a speech pathologist and a newly aphasic psychologist, the group continues to attract approximately 12 current and former in-patients for twice weekly sessions. Although attendance is optional for everyone, the outpatients, in particular, come because they want to. Between themselves, they form car-pools so that no one is stranded. As a group they discuss problems. Sometimes, they discuss the world problems, but most of the time they talk about shared personal concerns, like depression, sexual performance, financial insecurity, boredom, loss of self-esteem and family relationships. This, too, is a form of aphasia therapy. For patients who willingly drive 50 or more miles twice a week to attend such a group, it apparently is an effective one.

Conclusion

We have reviewed spontaneous recovery and efficacy of therapy in aphasia. We have suggested that the interactive nature of these two processes probably works for the benefit of the aphasic patient. We have further stated our belief that the rehabilitation of such patients shows positive effects long beyond the end of the period of spontaneous recovery. The most stringent tests of the efficacy of treatment, in fact, involve changes as a result of treatment in patients for whom spontaneous recovery itself is no longer an issue.

Finally, because the bulk of the literature indicates that treatment for aphasia is efficacious, we believe the stage has been set to begin the study of what forms of treatment work best with different types of aphasias and different aphasic people. This is the next step in the search for truly appropriate treatment strategies.

REFERENCES

Albert, M., Goodglass, H., Helm, N., Rubens, A., & Alexander, M. Clinical aspects of dysphasia. New York: Springer-Verlag, 1981.

Barresi, B., & Helm-Estabrooks, N. The Syntax Stimulation Program: A treatment approach for agrammatism. Presentation at American Speech, Language, Hearing Association. Los Angeles, November, 1981.

Basso, A., Faglioni, P., & Vignolo, L. Etude controlee de la reeducation du language dans l'aphasie: Comparison entre aphasiques traites et nontraites. Revue Neurologique (Paris), 1975, 131, 607-614.

Basso, A., Capitani, E., & Vignolo, L. Influence of rehabilitation on language skills in aphasic patients: A controlled study. Archives of Neurology, 1979, 36, 190-196.

Benson, D.F. Aphasia rehabilitation. Archives of Neurology, 1979, 36, 187-189.

Blair, J., Walsh, M., & Cerny, S. The group as an adjustment modality for aphasia patients. Presented to American Society for Group Psychotherapy and Psychodrama Annual Meeting. New York, April, 1979.

Brust, J., Shafer, S., Rechter, R., & Braun, B. Aphasia in acute stroke. Stroke, 1976, 7, 167-174.

Canter, G.J. Observations on neurogenic stuttering: A contribution to differential diagnosis. British Journal of Disorders of Communication, 1971, 6, 139-143.

Culton, G. Spontaneous recovery from aphasia. Journal of Speech and Hearing Research, 1969, 12, 825-832.

Demeurisse, G., Demol, O., Derouch, M., deBeucklaer, R., Coekaerts, M.J., & Capon, A. Quantitative study of the rate of recovery from aphasia due to ischemic stroke. Stroke, 1980, 11, 455-458.

Eisenson, J. Prognostic factors related to language rehabilitation in aphasic patients. Journal of Speech and Hearing Research, 1949, 14, 262-264.

Gleason, J.B., Goodglass, H., Green, E., Ackerman, N., & Hyde, M.K. The retrieval of syntax in Broca's aphasia. Brain and Language, 1975, 2, 451-471.

Goodglass, H., & Kaplan, E. Boston Diagnostic Aphasia Examination. Philadelphia: Lea & Febiger, 1972.

Helm-Estabrooks, N., Fitzpatrick, P., & Barresi, B. Response of an agrammatic patient to a syntax stimulation program for aphasia. Journal of Speech and Hearing Research, 1981, 46, 90-95.

Helm-Estabrooks, N., Fitzpatrick, P., & Barresi, B. Visual Action Therapy for global aphasia. Journal of Speech and Hearing Research, 1982, 47, 634-641.

Holland, A.L. The effectiveness of treatment for aphasia: A serendipitous study. In R. Brookshire (Ed.), Clinical aphasiology conference proceedings, 1980.

Holland, A.L. Communicative Abilities in Daily Living: A test of functional communication for aphasic adults. Baltimore, University Press, 1980.

Keenan, J., & Brassell, E. A study of factors related to prognosis for individual aphasic patients. Journal of Speech and Hearing Research, 1974, 39, 257-369.

Kenin, M., & Swisher, L. A study of pattern of recovery in aphasia. Cortex, 1972, 8, 56-68.

Kertesz, A., & McCabe, P. Recovery patterns and prognosis in aphasia. Brain, 1977, 100, 1-18.

Levita, E. Effects of speech therapy on aphasics' responses to the functional communication profile. Perceptual and Motor Skills, 1978, 47, 151-154.

Lomas, J., & Kertesz, A. Patterns of spontaneous recovery in aphasia groups: A study of adult stroke patients. Brain and Language, 1978, 5, 388-401.

Ludlow, C. Recovery from aphasia: A foundation for treatment. In M. Sullivan, & M. Kommens (Eds.), Rationale for adult aphasia therapy. Omaha: University of Nebraska Press, 1977.

Meier, M.J. Some challenges for clinical neuropsychology. In R. Reitan, & L. Davison (Eds.), Clinical neuropsychology, current status and applications. Washington, D.C.: Winston, 1974.

Mills, C.K. Treatment of aphasia by training. Journal of the American Medical Association, 1904, 43, 1940-1949.

Mohr, J.P. Rapid amelioration of motor aphasia. Archives of Neurology, 1973, 28, 77-82.

Porch, B.E. Porch Index of Communicative Ability. Palo Alto: Consulting Psychologists Press, 1971.

Porch, B., Collins, M., Wertz, R., & Fridan, T. Statistical prediction of change in aphasics. Journal of Speech and Hearing Research, 1980, 23, 312-321.

Pryse-Phillips, W. Rehabilitation of the patient with hemiplegia. In H.T. Conn (Ed.), Current therapy. Philadelphia: W.B.

Saunders Co., 1980.

Reinvang, I., & Engvik, H. Language recovery in aphasia from 3 to 6 months after stroke. In M.T. Sarno, & O. Hook (Eds.), Aphasia assessment and treatment. New York: Marson, 1980.

Riese, W. The early history of aphasia. Bulletin of the History of Medicine, 1947, 21, 322-334.

Rubens, A. The role of changes within the central nervous system during recovery from aphasia. In M. Sullivan, & M. Kommens (Eds.), Rationale for adult aphasia therapy. Omaha: University of Nebraska Press, 1977.

Sarno, M.T. The Functional Communication Profile. New York: Institute of Rehabilitation, New York University Medical Center, 1969.

Sarno, M.T., & Levita, E. Natural course of recovery in severe aphasia. Archives of Physical Medicine and Rehabilitation, 1971, 52, 175-179.

Sarno, M.T., & Levita, E. Recovery in treated aphasia in the first year post-stroke. Stroke, 1979, 10, 663-669.

Singer, H.D., & Low, A.A. The brain in the case of motor aphasia in which improvement occurred with training. Archives of Neurology and Psychiatry, 1933, 29, 162-165.

Sparks, R.W., Helm, N.A., & Albert, M. Aphasia rehabilitation resulting from melodic intonation therapy. Cortex, 1974, 10, 303-316.

Vignolo, L.A. Evolution of aphasia and language rehabilitation: A retrospective exploratory study. Cortex, 1964, 1, 344-367.

Wertz, R.T., Collins, M.J., Weiss, D., Kurtzke, J.F., Fridan, R., Brookshire, R.H., & Pierce, J. Veterans Administration cooperative study on aphasia: A comparison of individual and group treatment. Journal of Speech and Hearing Research, 1981, 24, 580-584.

Wertz, R.T., Kitselman, K.P., & Deal, L.A. Classifying the aphasias: Contributions to patient management. Presented to the annual meeting of the Academy of Apahsia. London, Ontario, 1981

Weisenburg, T.S., & McBride, K. Aphasia: A clinical and psychological study. New York: The Commonwealth Fund, 1935.

NEUROPSYCHOLOGICAL ASSESSMENT OF PSYCHIATRIC PATIENTS

Gerald Goldstein

Highland Drive Veterans Administration Medical Center
Pittsburgh, PA

The purpose of this chapter is that of providing a discussion of the role of neuropsychological testing in a psychiatric setting. Elsewhere (Goldstein, in press), we have described the contributions made by neuropsychology to the field of psychiatry in general, but here we wish to focus on just the matter of clinical assessment. The matter is a controversial one. Some neuropsychologists maintain the view that the standard neuropsychological tests were never intended to discriminate between "brain damaged" and "psychiatric" patients and it should not, therefore, be surprising when efforts at accomplishing this task fail to be successful. However, the practical reality seems to be that neuropsychologists work in psychiatric settings and are commonly asked to identify brain damaged patients within the context of a general neuropsychiatric population. Indeed, the term "neuropsychiatric" generally implies a mixed population of patients with a variety of functional psychiatric disorders, neurological disorders and mixtures of the two. The neurological patients generally tend to have chronic disorders, and differ substantially in many ways from the kinds of patients seen on acute neurology and neurosurgery wards.

Before getting into our topic directly, it may be worthwhile to describe such settings, and the distinctions between them and the acute neurology and neurosurgery facilities in which clinical neuropsychology was initially developed. Large neuropsychiatric hospitals generally provide facilities for short term care of acute psychiatric patients, long term care of mainly chronic schizophrenic patients and nursing home like care for patients in the end states of progressive dementing diseases. These institutions may also have outpatient clinics for ambulatory psychiatric patients and a number of special programs, particularly for alcoholic patients. Indeed,

many of the neuropsychological studies of chronic alcoholic Korsakoff's syndrome were accomplished in these settings. Thus, the emphasis tends to be on long term care of patients with usually very
chronic psychiatric and neurological disorders. In recent years
these institutions have largely been vacated by psychiatric patients
who moved back into the community, but the neurological patients,
particularly those with dementias, remain. It is apparent that this
type of population stands in sharp contrast to what is characteristic
of acute neurological and neurosurgical hospitals. These latter
facilities generally treat patients over a relatively short time
course and usually during the early stages of their illnesses. Thus,
for example, an individual who recently sustained a stroke would
typically be treated on an acute neurology ward and might later be
sent to a rehabilitation or convalescent facility for another relatively brief period of continued care. However, if the stroke gradually evolved into a multi-infarct dementia, the patient could eventually become hospitalized for a lengthy time period in a neuropsychiatric facility.

Neuropsychiatric facilities, as described above, typically employ clinical psychologists to assess and treat their patients, and
more recently have employed clinical neuropsychologists. During the
past, the clinical psychologists were frequently asked to test
patients for the purpose of contributing toward a differential diagnosis between a functional or organic condition. The methods used
to make these assessments were usually the standard psychological
tests of personality and intelligence. Sometimes, some of the early
appearing neuropsychological tests such as the Goldstein-Scheerer
tests and the Bender-Gestalt test were also used. For the most part,
the attempt was made to use these tests to discriminate between
chronically brain damaged and chronic schizophrenic patients. The
results of studies evaluating the capacity of neuropsychological
tests to make this discrimination and related ones have been thor-
ourghly reviewed in numerous places elsewhere and will not be repeated here (Malec, 1978; Goldstein, 1978; Heaton, Baade & Johnson,
1978; Heaton & Crowley, 1981). The general conclusion reached is
that while neuropsychological tests generally do discriminate between "functional" and "organic" disorders at psychometrically satisfactory levels, they do not do so in the case of chronic or process schizophrenia. Chronic process schizophrenics characteristically perform like brain damaged patients on these tests. We would
just emphasize the point that this conclusion has been extremely
well supported in numerous studies and, in our view, can be accepted
as a stable finding. However, the reason behind this finding is not
at all clear.

NEUROPSYCHOLOGY AND PSYCHOPATHOLOGY

The field of psychopathology as a scientific discipline has
historically encompassed many movements, schools and conceptual

frameworks. Typically, they have had their ascendance and decline, to be followed by newer, perhaps more innovative approaches. Even within certain types of psychopathology such as schizophrenia or the affective disorders, there have been countervailing theories and beliefs. While there are still many unanswered questions regarding psychopathology, it is generally felt that the role of theory generation has been productive, and has led to experimentation and clinical exploration that has increased scientific knowledge of the various mental disorders. However, much of the work in neuropsychological assessment of psychiatric patients has been atheoretical and at its worst, simply an attempt to take some single test and see if "organics" score differently on it from "schizophrenics" or some other group of psychiatric patients. The point we will try to develop here is that this excessive empiricism appears to have come up with very little, and that advances in neuropsychological assessment of psychiatric patients must await the development of some conceptual framework that allows investigators to generate some expectations of what they will find in their research. It now seems apparent that had these early investigators been aware of the literature concerning conceptual thinking deficits in schizophrenia and the bases for them, they would not have been at all surprised at the failure of complex cognitive tasks in discriminating between brain damaged patients and schizophrenics. Such a failure could have been readily hypothesized from what was known about cognition in schizophrenia.

There has been an interface between neuropsychology and psychopathology for some time, although it may not have been viewed as such in the past. For example, the Columbia-Greystone studies (Mettler, 1949) involved before and after cognitive testing of schizophrenic patients who underwent surgery or sham surgery on various sections of their frontal lobes. The use of cognitive tests, some of which are now known as neuropsychological tests, with psychiatric patients, goes back at least to the work of Rapaport (1945), who described the application of intelligence and sorting tests to assessment of psychiatric patients. Some neuropsychologists of the past, notably Kurt Goldstein and Martin Scheerer, did not make the sharp distinctions we now seem to make between brain damaged and psychiatric patients, and attempted to apply some general cognitive theory to both groups. For example, Goldstein and Scheerer's (1941) work stressed significance of impairment of the "abstract attitude" for both brain damaged and schizophrenic patients.

During recent years, there has been a renewed interest in the applications of neuropsychological methods to assessment of various forms of psychopathology. In our opinion, the major emphases have involved the following areas: (1) Schizophrenia; (2) Temporal Lobe Disorders; (3) Affective Disorders; (4) Psychiatric Conditions of the Elderly (Geropsychiatry): and, (5) Alcoholism. The remainder of this chapter will contain brief reviews of recent developments in these five broad areas, stressing clinical testing and application. Thus, for example, in the case of schizophrenia, issues raised will concern definition of the disorder, the nature of brain-behavior relationships specific to it and the state-of-the-art regarding evaluation of these relationships. It should be stated in advance that we are still a long way from resolving the current differential diagnosis difficulties, but we now have some interesting leads.

Schizophrenia. In essence, the major differential diagnostic problem regarding neuropsychological assessment of chronic schizophrenic patients is that many of them perform on the standard neuropsychological tests in a manner that is indistinguishable from that of patients with generalized, chronic brain disorders. This overlap is so pervasive that even when schizophrenic patients acquire structural brain damage through head injury, vascular disease or other processes, they cannot be distinguished from nonbrain damaged schizophrenics (Goldstein & Halperin, 1977). It appears that the cognitive deficits associated with the schizophrenia almost totally mask deficits that may be attributable to structural brain disorder. Data collected in our laboratory with the Halstead-Reitain battery attest to this difficulty. Table 1 contains means and standard deviations on the battery for groups of brain damaged schizophrenics, nonbrain damaged schizophrenics, brain damaged nonschizophrenics, and subjects who are neither brain damaged nor schizophrenic. Four group discriminant analysis initially classified subjects at a greater than chance level, but the "hit rate" was only 56.5% correct. On cross-validation, however, the hit-rate was reduced to 32%, a value that only minimally exceeds 25%, the chance expectation. Essentially, all of the subjects in this study were chronic patients, and so these data are quite consistent with what has been found by others (Heaton & Crowley, 1981).

It is possible that the reasons for this failure to discriminate are becoming clarified. Apparently, some of them are methodological in nature and some are substantive. The methodological problems resolve around issues of accuracy of diagnosis, effects of medication and other somatic therapies, and failure to adequately evaluate schizophrenic subjects for the presence of structural brain damage. The substantive problems are quite varied. First, and perhaps foremost, impressive data are accumulating indicating that a certain proportion of the schizophrenic population has clearly identifiable brain damage. While many investigators formerly speculated that this condition was the case, recently acquired CT scan and PETT scan evidence has confirmed the speculation with images of schizophrenic brains and measures of brain metabolism (Golden, Moses, Zelazowski, Graber, Zatz, Horvath, & Berger, 1980; Reider, Donnelly, Herdt, & Waldman, 1979). Neuropsychological studies done in conjunction with the CT scan studies found a significant degree of congruence between test performance and presence of atrophy noted on the scan. While the nature of this brain damage is not understood, its presence and its corres-

Table 1
Means and Standard Deviations of
Halstead-Reitan Battery Data

Variable	Brain Damaged Schizophrenic		Nonbrain Damaged Schizophrenic		Brain Damaged Schizophrenic		Nonbrain Damaged Schizophrenic	
	M	SD	M	SD	M	SD	M	SD
WAIS Subtests (Scaled Scores)								
Information	9.98	2.23	10.24	2.52	9.74	3.65	10.38	2.45
Comprehension	9.96	2.22	10.18	3.84	9.64	3.84	11.18	3.04
Arithmetic	9.94	3.03	9.22	3.49	8.40	3.66	10.12	2.85
Similarities	9.16	2.36	10.02	3.01	9.52	4.31	9.92	3.30
Digit Span	8.82	2.57	9.10	3.14	8.82	3.53	9.70	2.35
Vocabulary	9.54	1.94	10.30	3.03	10.00	3.65	10.36	2.82
Digit Symbol	6.48	2.85	6.82	2.68	5.48	2.86	7.92	2.27
Picture Completion	8.84	2.60	8.88	2.54	8.22	3.25	9.54	2.79
Block Design	8.20	2.71	8.64	3.13	7.88	3.29	9.10	2.94
Picture Arrangement	7.82	1.86	7.80	2.52	6.88	2.73	8.70	2.28
Object Assembly	8.30	2.79	9.04	3.02	7.70	3.16	9.52	3.22
Other Measures								
NTD Seconds	9.40	4.23	8.70	3.11	10.72	5.51	7.90	3.38
NTN Seconds	22.38	9.94	22.58	11.68	26.22	11.59	19.84	9.51
TVD Seconds	8.14	4.66	6.64	2.79	8.78	5.70	6.32	2.53
TVND Seconds	14.86	6.61	13.54	4.72	17.28	8.12	13.38	4.74
GRD Kgm	38.68	10.84	39.40	11.72	36.44	11.43	38.60	12.49
GRND Kgm	37.32	10.28	37.04	10.93	32.78	10.48	35.76	13.25
HCT Errors	71.14	28.16	77.56	34.33	87.42	32.77	67.52	31.18
TPT-T Minutes	22.67	6.60	19.63	6.87	23.31	6.72	18.23	6.91
TPT-M #Blocks	6.34	2.29	5.82	2.12	5.52	2.41	6.28	2.26

Table 1 (Cont'd)

Variable	Brain Damaged Schizophrenic		Nonbrain Damaged Schizophrenic		Brain Damaged Schizophrenic		Nonbrain Damaged Schizophrenic	
	M	SD	M	SD	M	SD	M	SD
TPT-L #Blocks	2.32	2.51	2.64	2.27	2.06	2.24	2.92	2.20
SP Errors	13.26	8.35	10.24	7.51	13.22	9.41	10.60	6.70
RHY Errors	7.28	3.80	7.94	4.84	8.54	4.54	7.22	3.88
TRA Seconds	47.60	30.31	45.46	25.92	63.88	45.32	34.40	11.64
TRB Seconds	127.80	61.28	140.20	101.49	172.68	86.21	96.78	55.67
TAPD #/10 Sec.	41.34	9.39	44.72	10.59	38.44	10.82	46.32	9.42
TAPN #/10 Sec.	37.56	9.66	40.04	8.50	34.84	9.41	40.98	7.69
APH Errors	8.74	5.48	7.14	6.08	9.88	7.31	5.54	4.07
PD	20.62	15.96	16.10	13.12	22.32	16.41	12.28	10.37
No. of Cases	50		50		50		50	

Note. Other measures: NTD = Name Time, Dominant Hand; NTN = Name time, Nondominant Hand;

TVD = TV Time, Dominant Hand; TVND = TV Time, Nondominant Hand; GRD = Grip, Nondominant Hand,

HCT = Halstead Category Test; TPT-T = Tactual Performance Test (Time); TPT-M = Tactual Per-

formance Test (Memory); TPT-L = Tactual Performance Test (Location); SP = Speech Perception;

RHY = Rhythm Test; TRA = Trail Making, Part A; TRB = Trail Making, Part B; TAPD = Tapping,

Dominant Hand; TAPN = Tapping, Nondominant Hand; APH = Aphasia Test; PD = Perceptual Disorders.

pondence with impairment of higher brain functions provide some verification to the often stated view that some schizophrenics look
brain damaged on cognitive tests because they are brain damaged.
However, the issue is more complicated than that as we will see.

One apparent problem is that it would appear to be quite difficult at present to relate what is known about the clinical phenomenology of schizophrenia to these changes in brain structure. That
is, the brain abnormalities noted do not appear to contribute to a
further understanding of such phenomena as delusions, hallucinations,
autism and other common manifestations of the schizophrenic process.
A related matter has to do with whether or not the amount of structural brain damage noted is congruent with the degree of cognitive
impairment. Still another issue revolves around the commonly held
view that schizophrenia is not a single entity, but a variety of
disorders. Do all schizophrenics have these brain abnormalities or
are they found only in certain subtypes? These considerations and
others have elicited more detailed investigations of brain structure
and function in schizophrenic patients.

There appears to be a general consensus that somehow the schizophrenic, or the schizophrenic brain, processes information differently from normal. A major current hypothesis concerning this difference relates to cerebral hemisphere asymmetries, with most investigators suggesting that schizophrenics process information in a defective manner with their left or dominant cerebral hemispheres
(Gruzelier & Flor-Henry, 1979). There are several versions of this
basic hypothesis, but in general, the left hemisphere is implicated.
The dysfunction has been noted at the psychophysiological level
(Gruzelier, 1979), the sensory-motor level (Gur, 1978), and the cognitive level (Gordon, Goldstein, & Sabol, 1982). Luchins, Weinberger,
& Wyatt (1979) even suggest the presence of a neuroanatomic analog
of this asymmetry in the form of a reversal of the normal asymmetry
of the brain as seen on the CT scan. Some schizophrenics show a
reversal from the normal relationship in which the right frontal lobe
is wider than the left, and the left occipital lobe is wider than
the right. With regard to brain function, cerebral blood flow and
PETT scan data (Ingvar, Brun, Hagberg, & Gustafson, 1978; Buchsbaum,
1981), have shown abnormal patterns among schizophrenics. Electrophysiological data suggest that the schizophrenic patient does not
develop a normal visual evoked potential, particularly in regard to
the late components of the wave from (P300) (Levit, Sutton, & Zubin,
1973). In summary, there is abundant evidence for deviations from
normal in the structure and function of the schizophrenic brain.
Thus, early attempts at discriminating between "brain damage" and
"schizophrenia" may, in retrospect, be viewed as somewhat naive.

If it is assumed that schizophrenia is indeed a form of brain
dysfunction, then the nature of clinical assessment should change
from what it was in the past. In the past, it seemed to be assumed

that although the schizophrenic patient looked like the brain damaged patient on tests, the similarity was superficial. The brain
damaged patient was seen as demonstrating impairment because of an
inability to perform the task, while the schizophrenic was viewed
as a patient who really could perform the task but failed to do so
because of difficulties with maintaining attention, interference by
intruding thoughts or failure of motivation. This view, in the light
of current theory and evidence, would now also be viewed as somewhat
naive or simplistic. A commonly accepted approach in contemporary
psychopathology and neuropsychology involves an application of information theory, and an analysis of various neuropsychological and
psychopathological syndromes in terms of information processing
deficits (Kietzman, Sutton, & Zubin, 1975). In schizophrenia, there
is thought to be some breakdown in the normal process of getting
information into and through the central nervous system and it is
this breakdown that is felt to have a strong relationship to the apparent symptoms or clinical phenomenology of the disorder. Some investigators are interested in these phenomena at a purely behavioral
level, although they grant the possibility of some defect in the
physiological substrate, while others, notably neuropsychologists,
maintain a strong, direct interest in the physiological substrate.
Among this latter group, there is currently a great deal of interest
in cerebral hemisphere asymmetries and the idea that schizophrenics
have defective left hemisphere function. In information processing
terms, there are various ways in which this phenomenon may be expres-
sed. At the cognitive level, it can be said that schizophrenics
attempt to apply "right hemisphere strategies" or methods involving
global, synthetic processing to tasks better dealt with through "left
hemisphere" or analytic, sequential strategies. An alternative view,
one proposed by Gur (1978) is that schizophrenics overactivate their
defective left hemisphere, or attempt to apply defective "left hemisphere" processes ineffectively, since the capacity to utilize those
processes is impaired. In a similar vein, Magaro (1978) has proposed
that paranoids overutilize controlled processing, a sequential, "left
hemisphere" strategy, while nonparanoid schizophrenics overutilize
automatic processing, a perceptually oriented "right hemisphere" form
of processing information. Data obtained in our own laboratory
(Gordon, Goldstein, & Sabol, 1982) suggest that schizophrenics do
better at "right hemisphere cognitive tasks" (i.e., tasks requiring
perception of gestalts and synthesis) than at "left hemisphere tasks"
(those requiring analysis and sequencing).

    Along with, or in spite of, these recent developments in psy-
chopathology, the standard neuropsychological tests continue to be
administered in clinical practice, often with the aim of providing
information to "rule out organicity." Indeed, the Luria-Nebraska
neuropsychological battery has recently been studied in reference
to just this matter (Purisch, Golden, & Hammeke, 1978). This battery of tests, consisting of a selection of items developed by
Luria and his co-workers for neuropsychological assessment of brain

damaged patients, was found to have 88% diagnostic accuracy with regard to discriminating between a sample of schizophrenics and a sample of patients with miscellaneous forms of structural brain damage. While the brain damaged patients did poorly on items involving both simple perceptual and motor functions and complex cognitive functions, the schizophrenics only did poorly on the items involving complex functions. In information processing terms, these results might suggest that while brain damaged patients have difficulties in the sensory, perceptual and cognitive information processing domains, schizophrenics have their major difficulty in the cognitive domain, with relative sparing of basic sensory and perceptual processes. However, such an inference may be premature, since the Luria-Nebraska items were not subjected to an information processing analysis, which requires the sequential tracing of events from stimulus input through central mediation processes to response. Furthermore, because of methodological problems often associated with research in schizophrenia (Heaton & Crowley, 1981; Goldstein, 1978), and with the Luria-Nebraska battery (Adams, 1980), it is somewhat difficult to interpret these findings. Nevertheless, the matter of dissociation between simpler perceptual and motor processes as opposed to complex processes may be of substantial significance for differential diagnosis.

The failure of much of the differential diagnosis research in regard to discrimination between brain damaged and schizophrenic patients with neuropsychological tests may now be viewed less as a disappointment and more as a set of uninterpretable findings. The major difficulty seems to be that in the absence of the new brain imaging technology, which was not available at the time of much of this research, it was not possible to determine how many of the schizophrenic subjects had brain atrophy or other structural anomalies such as an enlarged corpus callosum (Rosenthal & Bigelow, 1972) or reversed asymmetry (Luchins, Weinberger, & Wyatt, 1979). Thus, a number of the "schizophrenic" subjects in these studies may well have had structural impairment of brain substance comparable in nature and degree to what was the case for the "brain damaged" subjects. The availability of the CT scan may assist substantially in resolving this particular problem in diagnostic evaluation. It is possible, but not proven, that the standard neuropsychological tests were doing their job all the time with schizophrenic patients, but what they were doing was providing a behavioral index of the degree of loss of brain substance; exactly what they are supposed to do.

Perhaps it is useful to make a distinction between neuropsychological assessment in a neuropsychiatric setting, in which the diagnostician is confronted with the practical task of appropriate and useful assessment and classification, and the more basic matter of the neuropsychology of schizophrenia. The former problem area has traditionally been viewed as belonging in the realm of psychometrics, the research effort involving the development of valid and reliable

instruments. The latter area has been the subject of a great deal
of theoretically oriented experimental research. Psychometric studies have been persistently confounded by methodological problems too
numerous to mention here. As an example, Heaton and Crowley's (1981)
list includes (1) failures in proper sampling methodology; (2) failures in describing the bases for psychiatric diagnoses; (3) failure
to adequately document neurological diagnoses; (4) failure to rule
out neurological disorder in the psychiatric group; (5) failure to
report or control for chronicity of illness; (6) failure to equate
groups for age and education; (7) inappropriate matching of subjects
for IQ; (8) failure to report or control for somatic therapies. On
the other hand, the experimental research in schizophrenia has not
arrived at anything approaching a commonly accepted theory, but
rather has gotten into what Zubin and Steinhauer (1981) describe as
a logjam; a mass of data and a plethora of theories that appear to
be impeding further progress. The problems here are not primarily
methodological in that the methodology and design of many contemporary studies of schizophrenia are quite elegant, but have more to do
with the lack of a unifying theory that integrates the masses of
data coming from a variety of disciplines. Zubin and Steinhauer
(1981) adopt a vulnerability model as a proposed solution, but we
will not elaborate on or attempt to evaluate that proposal here.
The point is that both psychometric and theoretical experimental
research in the area of schizophrenia continue to have to deal with
a number of unresolved issues, and the need for further research is
apparent.

    With regard to the matter of neuropsychological assessment, the
following tentative conclusions can be reached. There is evidence
coming from two laboratories that some schizophrenic patients have
demonstrable brain atrophy and that the degree of atrophy is associated with extent of neuropsychological impairment. As a screening
assessment procedure, there is evidence from a single laboratory
that the Luria-Nebraska battery may provide more accurate discrimination between brain damaged and schizophrenic patients than does the
Halstead-Reitan battery. However, because of numerous methodological problems and the absence of a direct Luria-Nebraska vs. Halstead-
Reitan comparison with the same sample, this conclusion has to be
very tentative. There is evidence coming from many settings that a
specific neuropsychological deficit in schizophrenia is some form
of dysfunction of the left cerebral hemisphere. The dysfunction
is seen in psychophysiological responsivity, lateral eye movements
and cognitive function. Among those that agree that some functional
deviation from normal in regard to cerebral hemisphere asymmetries
is important for the understanding of schizophrenia, several theoretical formulations have emerged in attempts to explain the phenomenon. The whole matter of abnormal hemisphere asymmetries in psychopathology is currently undergoing intensive investigation.

    As a concluding comment, we would add that the task remains of bridging the gap between psychometric and experimental findings on the one hand and descriptive psychopathology on the other. We may be reminded that the clinical phenomenology of schizophrenia involves delusions, auditory hallucinations, loosening of associations, and flat or inappropriate affect. It is the hope of neuropsychologists and those interested in information processing that the relatively subtle cognitive and perceptual deficits noted in their evaluations are associated with these more blatant symptoms. In this regard, Kietzman, Spring and Zubin (1980) made the following pertinent remarks concerning laboratory studies of schizophrenia:

> Often those studies seem rather arid and removed from meaningful contexts in the lives of psychiatric patients. In fact, one often wonders why those investigations were ever begun, since they seem to reveal deviant responses far removed from those presented as the patient's chief complaint. It is the authors' premise here that the deviant responses patients display in laboratory testing underlie some of the symptoms they present clinically.

The Temporal Lobes and Psychiatric Disorder. The temporal lobes are complex structures involved in mediating a number of functions including hearing, memory, language and visual perception. However, we will only be concerned here with those phenomena associated with temporal lobe dysfunction that look "psychiatric" in nature. By this colloquialism we simply mean those disorders of temporal lobe function that give rise to the kinds of symptoms more frequently seen in patients with functional psychiatric disorders; most typically the schizophrenic and affective disorders. Generally, these phenomena are diagnosed as complex partial seizures or temporal lobe epilepsy, and the symptoms may include visual hallucinations, illusions giving the appearance of objects being larger or smaller than they are, olfactory hallucinations, depersonalization experiences, deja vu and jamais vu experiences and episodes of purposive looking but bizarre behavior. The latter symptoms apparently gave rise to the term "psychomotor epilepsy" which is still sometimes used to describe this condition.

Beyond the matter of assessment and treatment of patients with temporal lobe epilepsy, the study of these disorders has provided a number of significant hypotheses concerning important neurological mechanisms in schizophrenia and the affective disorders. Indeed, Flor-Henry and Yeudall's (1979) early explorations with temporal lobe epileptics led directly to the work with hemiphere asymmetries in schizophrenia. Moreover, this work was also associated with the corrollary hypothesis that the affective disorders bore some relationship to dysfunction of the right temporal lobe. From relatively early in the history of psychiatry, it was thought that some anomaly in brain structure or function provided the basis for some of the major psychiatric disorders. The original rationles for such somatic therapies as psychosurgery and electroconvulsive therapy were essentially based on that belief. Parallels have been drawn between the ictal behavior of temporal lobe epileptics and schizophrenic symptomatology. Altered states of consciousness and the development of hallucinations are commonly seen in both conditions. The crucial set of structures in all of these matters appears to be the limbic system, the portion of the brain that appears to be highly associated with mediation of the emotions. Gruzelier (1979) has, in fact, made the strong suggestion that the left temporal lobe and underlying limbic system may be the areas that are responsible for several of the cardinal symptoms of schizophrenia. Discussions of this hypothesis are provided throughout Gruzelier and Flor-Henry's (1979) text and in Boller, Detre and Kim (in press). Obviously, the hypothesis is a controversial and intriguing one.

Neuropsychological assessment of temporal lobe disorders is a complex matter because of the variety of functions in which the temporal lobes play a role. The only issue to be dealt with here relates to assessment of those patients with temporal lobe disease who present with the kinds of "psychiatric" symptomatology described above. The matter is complicated by the fact that there are major behavioral differences associated with the source of the temporal lobe dysfunction. Klove and Matthews (1974) report that patients with psychomotor (temporal lobe) epilepsy of unknown etiology show minimal if any deficit on the standard clinical neuropsychological tests. However, as is well known, patients with temporal lobe lesions of known etiology such as penetrating head wounds or focal vascular lesions may show prominent neuropsychological deficit in numerous areas including memory, language and visual or auditory perception (Walsh, 1978). In the case of the patient with temporal lobe epilepsy of unknown etiology, it is not unusual to see episodes involving hallucinations, automatic behavior, illusions and related phenomena, with no evidence of neuropsychological deficit during interictal periods.

There has been some investigation of the interictal behavior of temporal lobe epilepsy patients, the most well known study being by Bear and Fedio (1977). These investigators reported finding personality differences depending upon the side of the temporal lobe abnormality. Subjects with left temporal lobe epilepsy were reported as feeling more depressed than the right temporal cases, who in fact denied such feelings. The right temporals displayed greater affect than the lefts, while the lefts seemed more preoccupied with religious and moral ideation. There is also a fairly extensive literature, as indicated above, in which parallels are drawn between schizophrenia and temporal lobe epilepsy, but Bear and Fedio (1977) suggest that there are also striking differences between schizophrenics and temporal lobe epileptics including such matters as the deepened, as opposed to flattened, affect seen in temporal lobe epileptics, as well as their tendency to preserve social relations.

We will attempt to illustrate the controversies and complexities of the area of temporal lobe epilepsy with the following case illustration. The patient was a thirty year old man whose major presenting complaint was recurrent episodes of uncontrollable, violent behavior. The course of these episodes typically started with the onset of a headache. It would be followed by feelings of depression and anxiety with no apparent cause. On some occasions he developed blurred or double vision, and then would have a feeling of light headedness; as if walking on water. Then he would have the impulse to hit someone or something. He becomes amnesic for the remainder of the episode following this point, but based on observation of one of them while he was hospitalized, his face flushed, he began perspiring and his right arm became tremulous. He then seemed confused and asked to be restrained or locked up. He was placed in a locked room and while there banged his fist repeatedly into a wall to the extent that he slightly injured himself. The episode lasted about fifteen minutes, following which he felt tired, but was unable to recall what had occurred.

Is this temporal lobe epilepsy? The question turned out to be extremely diffcult to answer. The patient has a history of convulsions associated with high fever at 11 months of age. He also had hepatitis at age 11. He is a Viet Nam era veteran, and the records appear to clearly establish that he was exposed to the defoliant "Agent Orange." He was in combat, and sustained a leg wound. It is reported that he may also have sustained a "concussion" at the same time. According to the patient's mother, he underwent a personality change following his return from Viet Nam. Prior to then, there were none of the episodes of violence. To the contrary, he was described as friendly and even tempered, with no tendency toward impulsiveness. Following his return from Viet Nam, he was described as having an increasingly bad temper, with a tendency to "fly off the handle" at the slightest provocation. Psychiatric evaluations during this period, while noting the possibility of psychomotor epilepsy, also recognized his emotional problems and described them in terms of anxiety, depression and passive aggressive personality features. There seemed little question that the patient was having severe psychiatric difficulties. The major issue was the role of possible brain dysfunction in their etiology.

In view of the patient's complex history, he was given an extensive evaluation. A special physical examination was given designed to evaluate individuals who may have been exposed to toxic chemicals (Agent Orange in this case). It was noted that he had multiple skin abnormalities including multiple pigmented moles over

his body, punctate lesions on his thighs and a patchy macular rash
from the waist down. His physical neurological examination was reported as within normal limits, with no positive findings. A static
brain scan was reported as normal but cerebral blood flow studies
resulted in the finding of a failure to visualize the superior sag-
gital sinus. The possibility of an epidural hematoma was suggested,
but the skull X-Ray and CT scan were entirely normal, and the possibilities of an epidural or chronic subdural hematoma were ruled out.
Several EEGs were administered, the first one available to us being
done during 1973, about eight years before we evaluated him. It was
reported as normal. Two abnormal EEGs were obtained during March and
April of 1980. The first of them was marked by focal 3 to 4 cycles
per second slowing in both occipital regions, while the second one
contained low voltage fast activity in all leads. Another EEG, done
with nasopharyngeal leads during June of 1980 was read as normal.

The patient was administered two full neuropsychological test
batteries: the Halstead-Reitan and the Luria-Nebraska battery.
Quantitative results for these procedures are presented in Table 2.
As would be expected on the basis of the literature, the patient had
essentially no neuropsychological deficits. The only slightly sus-
picious findings involved his minimally impaired performance on the
Expressive Speech and Writing Scales of the Luria-Nebraska and the
discrepancy between verbal and performance WAIS IQs, with verbal
being lower than performance. Apparently, the patient has some
degree of difficulty with language, despite his high school level
education. It may also be noted in Table 2 that he performed in the
mid 6th grade level range on the Reading and Spelling sections of
the Wide Range Achievement Test. In view of the absence of neurological and neuropsychological evidence of structural brain damage,
it would seem most conservative to interpret these findings on a
developmental basis rather than in terms of adult acquired brain
damage.

While the diagnosis of temporal lobe epilepsy could never be
documented with certainty, the patient's physician nevertheless pre-
scribed anticonvulsant medication for him; Mysoline, 250mg in the
morning and 375mg at bedtime. This medication was given in combination with Cafergot, with instructions to take two tablets at the
onset of a headache, and Mellaril, 50mg to be taken as needed every
four hours during periods of tension. It was noted that the Cafergot
was very effective in regard to arresting the development of headaches. This combination of medications not only helped alleviate
the headaches, but the number of outbursts was also substantially
reduced. Unfortunately, because of the fact that the patient received a combination of medications, it is not possible to say
which one was most instrumental in reducing the number of episodes.
However, it is unlikely to be the Mellaril, since it was only used
on a very intermittent basis. One possibility is that, since the
episodes generally proceeded from a migraine type headache, the

Table 2.   Neuropsychological Test Data

Wechsler Adult Intelligence Scale		Halstead-Reitan Battery	
Information	10	Category Test	71 errors
Comprehension	9	Tactual Performance	
Arithmetic	11	Test-Time	9.7 minutes
Simlarities	13	Memory	9 blocks
Digit Span	7	Location	6 blocks
Vocabulary	8	Speech Perception	14 errors
Digit Symbol	11	Rhythm	5 errors
Picture Completion	12	Trailmaking	
Block Design	10	A	20 seconds
Picture Arrangement	9	B	39 seconds
Object Assembly	15	Finger Tapping	
Verbal IQ	97	R Hand	46 taps
Performance IQ	110	C Hand	40 taps
Full Scale IQ	103	Aphasic Screening	5 errors
		Average Impairment	
		& Rating = 1.00	
		% of Ratings in Impaired	
		Range = 25%	

Luria - Nebraska Battery

Scale	T	Scale	T
Motor	35	Reading	55
Rhythm	40	Arithmetic	40
Kinesthesis	44	Memory	38
Visual	35	IQ	55
Receptive Speech	42	Pathogonmonic	43
Expressive Speech	63	Right Hemisphere	43
Writing	63	Left Hemisphere	35

action of the Cafergot in regard to arresting the further development of the headache may be a very important factor.

This case was presented in some detail not because of its particular uniqueness but because of its representativeness. In our
experience, there appear to be many patients who have ictal episodes
that appear to be not inconsistent with psychomotor epilepsy, but
that do not meet rigorous diagnostic criteria. Bear and Fedio's
(1977) cases all had unilateral spike foci in the temporal lobes
and observed psychomotor seizures, but there appear to be a good
number of patients who have what look like temporal lobe seizures,
but who do not have the appropriate EEG abnormality. In this case,
there were several abnormal EEGs, but the abnormalities did not
consist of temporal lobe spikes. The patient demonstrated several
of the manifestations generally associated with complex partial
seizures including the sudden onset of severe anxiety, postictal
amnesia, rapid autonomic changes, and possibly the arm jerking and
face twitching. In view of this combination of symptoms without
definitive neurological documentation, the patient received a number
of psychiatric diagnoses including hysterical neurosis; conversion
type, passive-aggressive personality with hysterical features and
situational reaction with anxiety and depression. One examining
neurologist explicity stated that the patient had no neurological
disease and that he was one of the 10-15% of normal people with abnormal EEGs. It is not our intention here to declare that this
patient actually did or did not have epilepsy, but simply to point
out some of the diagnostic difficulties in this area. The fact that
there is some evidence that the patient's symptoms may have been
reduced by medication with anticonvulsant and anti-migraine medication may provide some evidence for an organic basis for his disorder,
but the complexities of many medications often make it very hazardous
to diagnose from drug response.

With regard to the matter of assessment of patients for temporal lobe epilepsy we may expect to find relatively normal performance on the standard neuropsychological tests, behavioral differences during interictal periods depending on whether the focus is
in the right or left temporal lobe and interictal symptomatology
that bears some resemblance, perhaps of a superficial nature, to
what is often seen in schizophrenic patients. Indeed, the term
"epileptic psychosis" has been used to describe this phenomenon
(Stevens, 1966). The point we wish to raise with our case example
is that the neuropsychologist working in a psychiatric settings, as
opposed to an epilepsy clinic, may see a number of patients with
presenting symptoms which may or may not be associated with docu-
mentable temporal lobe dysfunction. Such patients may produce normal results on clinical neuropsychological tests, and in fact may
have no specific abnormalities of any type associated with brain
dysfunction. Probably the best conclusion that can be reached about
these cases is that the current state-of-the-art does not permit the

establishment of a definitive diagnosis. It is, therefore, probably
best not to rule out any possibility particularly since, as in the
present case, these patients may respond favorably to being treated
as if they were epileptics.

    The Affective Disorders. It seems appropriate to present a
section on the temporal lobes between one on schizophrenia and another on the affective disorders, since the temporal lobes in general and the limbic system in particular, may have a great deal to
do with the etiology of both of these major classes of psychiatric
disorder. With regard to the affective disorders there are two
major issues; the neuropsychology of affect and the performance of
patients with affective disorders on standard neuropsychological
tests. In other words, how does the brain mediate affect and how
do extreme affective states affect performance in the cognitive and
perceptual spheres? The study of the physiology of the emotions has
a long history, going back at least to William James (James, 1890)
and through the contributions of such pioneers as Bard (1934) and
Cannon (1925; 1927). A brief review of this history traced to current thinking is contained in Valenstein and Heilman (1979). Important developments include the discovery of the limbic system and the
"Papez circuit" as mediators of emotion, the establishment of the
special role of the hypothalamus in regulation of the emotions, the
formulation of the place of the frontal lobes in controlling emotional
behavior and the discovery of hemisphere asymmetries in emotional
response.

    In recent years, the theory has emerged that at least some in-
dividuals with affective disorders may have lateralized neuropsychological dysfunction just as some patients with lateralized brain
lesions acquire characteristic affective disorders (Gainotti, 1972).
Flor-Henry and Yeudall (1979), and those who pursued the theory, have
suggested a parallel between the lateralized dysfunction of the left
hemisphere found in schizophrenic patients and a right hemisphere
defect in patients with depression. Indeed, a literature has developed suggesting the presence of right hemisphere deficit in clinically
depressed patients (Bruder & Yozawitz, 1979; Goldstein, Filskov,
Weaver, & Ives, 1977; Kronfol, Hamsher, Digre, & Waziri, 1978).
Some degree of backup from these findings has come from EEG and
evoked potential data, suggesting hypoarousal of the right hemisphere
in depressed patients (D'Elia & Perris, 1973, 1974; Perris & Monakhov, 1979). Several of the studies cited above looked at the effects
of ECT, with the general finding that there was an improvement in
right hemisphere function following ECT. We know of no comparable
studies involving the use of pharmacological agents.

    With regard to the matter of neuropsychological assessment,
there have been a variety of findings regarding patients with affective disorders. Utilizing a modified version of the Halstead-
Reitan battery, Flor-Henry and Yeudall (1979) found the expected

dominant hemisphere dysfunction for schizophrenics, but they also
found what they interpreted as primarily right hemisphere (nondominant) dysfunction in their manic-depressive group. The patients
who were manic fell between the schizophrenics and depressives in
some respects. This finding was particularly notable on a strength
of grip measure using a hand dynamometer. The asymmetry between
right and left hand was most pronounced in the schizophrenia group,
inbetween in the mania group and least in the depressive group. As
indicated above, other studies (Goldstein et al., 1977; Kronfol
et al., 1978) have also suggested primarily right hemisphere dysfunction in depressives. However, when one compares mixed groups of
patients with known structural brain damage with affective disorder
patients, neuropsychological tests generally make a reasonably good
discrimination. Heaton and Crowley (1981) reviewed 10 attempts to
classify subjects into "organic" and "mixed affective disorder"
groups and found that the mean "hit rate" was 77%; a reasonably
satisfactory result. He also notes an additional study by Watson,
Davis and Gasser (1978) in which depressives and brain damaged
patients were compared. Here, there were 83% correct classifications.
In summary, while some studies claim to have identified specific
right hemisphere dysfunction in depressed patients, other studies
have shown that depressed patients generally perform sufficiently
better than brain damaged patients to allow for psychometrically
satisfactory classificatory accuracy. While these findings are not
necessarily mutually contradictory, clarification is obviously required. It is possible that depressed individuals, in a manner of
speaking, prefer to process information with their left hemispheres,
but the possible deficiency upon which this preference may be based
is not at all comparable in extent to what is typically found in
individuals with known brain lesions. If this situation is the
case, then the depressed patient may be more accurately described
in terms of an extreme cognitive style than in terms of the way in
which patients with structural right hemisphere brain damage are
typically described.

     The above considerations may be associated in some way with a
severity dimension. Some physically healthy but mildly depressed
individuals might show essentially no neuropsychological deficit,
while more severely depressed individuals may. Many clinicians
might suspect that the presence of moderate to severe depression
might wreak havoc with neuropsychological test performance simply
because of the nature of the clinical phenomenology of depression.
In actuality, this belief is not confirmed by empirical studies in
which degree of depression was correlated with extent of neuropsychological deficit. Heaton and Crowley (1981) also reviewed this
matter and made the following concluding statement:

               The bulk of evidence presented in this
               section suggests that for most psychiatric
               patient groups there is little or no rela-

tionship between the degree of emotional disturbance and level of
performance on neuropsychological
tests.

In studies that specifically evaluated depressives, this conclusion
obtained particularly well. Perkins (1974) found no association
between degree of depression and score on the Halstead Category
Test. Friedman (1964) also noted the absence of correlations between a battery of ability tests and self or psychiatrist ratings
of degree of depression. Squire, Slater and Chace (1975) found no
relationship between degree of depression and performance on memory
tests. These findings would suggest that if a depressed patient
demonstrates deficits on neuropsychological tests, there is a strong
likelihood that the deficit is not based on the symptoms of the depression but either on unrelated brain damage or on some neuropsychological characteristic that may underlie at least certain types
of depression, such as right hemisphere temporal-limbic dysfunction.

It may be noted that we have not addressed ourselves to the
problem of reactive or secondary depression as seen in physical or
other psychiatric illness. The findings here are quite different
from those reviewed above in that there are substantial correlations
between degree of depression and extensiveness of neuropsychological
deficit in these cases. This matter has been studied for numerous
disease entities including Huntington's disease (Boll, Heaton, &
Reitan, 1974), aphasia (Dikmen & Reitan, 1974), and multiple sclerosis (Matthews, Cleeland, & Hopper, 1970). Furthermore, we have not
yet discussed the matter of depression in elderly patients when there
is a question of dementia, but will do so in our section on geriatric
psychiatry. Here, we were concerned with patients whose primary diagnosis is an affective disorder of the major recurrent or bipolar
type. In other words, these are individuals who have mood disturbances that are not produced by any other physical or mental disorder. In summarizing the neuropsychological assessment research done
with such patients, it might be fair to say that there has been a
reasonably solid and a more tentative conclusion drawn. The relatively solid conclusion is that neuropsychological tests discriminate reasonably well between depressed patients and patients with
structural brain damage. Furthermore, degree of depression is not
associated with level of neuropsychological test performance. The
more tentative finding is that at least some depressed individuals
have right hemisphere dysfunction comparable to the left hemisphere
dysfunction found in some schizophrenics. Further investigation of
this matter is needed because of the relatively small number of
studies in which clearly positive findings were obtained, the tendency in these studies to go beyond the data in terms of definition
of right hemisphere neuropsychological functions and other methodological problems. It is particularly important to note that the
speed component of many visual-spatial, so-called, "right hemisphere"

tests may introduce a general efficiency factor sensitive to damage
to any area of the brain. Many "right hemisphere" tests also tend
to be more complex and difficult than "left hemisphere" tests,
since they often require adaptive complex problem solving ability
as opposed to simple retrieval of overlearned material. Thus, in
the case of the neuropsychological aspects of depression, it is
particularly important to assure oneself that right hemisphere functions are in fact relatively impaired, and that we are not looking
at the tendency of depressed individuals to do less well at timed,
novel tasks than at tasks only requiring retrieval processes from
long term storage.

Geropsychiatry: Psychiatric Disorders of the Elderly. Most
clinicians would probably agree that the major psychiatric disorders
of the elderly are dementia, depression and stresses that derive
from impaired cognitive and sensory function that are not sufficiently
severe to be classified as a dementia or other disorder of the central nervous system. As an example of the latter point, we have
the "benign senescent forgetfulness" described by Kral (1978). This
condition is characterized as the inability to recall unimportant
data or parts of an experience, although the experience itself can
be recalled. Furthermore, the material that cannot be recalled on
one occasion, such as a name, a place or a date, can be recalled at
some other time. The term "benign" is used in opposition to the so-
called "malignant" amnesic syndromes. Kral (1978) found that there
were striking differences in death rate and survival time between
elderly individuals with "benign" and "malignant" disorders. While
impairment of memory may be benign when defined in this manner, it
may nevertheless be stressful and discomforting. Individuals with
this condition are said to be quite aware of it and may be apolo-
getic for their forgetfulness, or may attempt to compensate for it
through circumlocution.

A challenge to the diagnostic accuracy and thus the usefulness
of neuropsychological testing with the elderly has been issued by
Wells (1980). Following some complimentary remarks concerning the
efficacy of neuropsychological tests in assessment of cerebral function, he adds the following sentences:

> Such findings do not, however, demonstrate,
> in patients whose diagnosis is uncertain,
> that neuropsychological testing can pre-
> dictably identify which patient has organic
> disease and which does not. When the prob-
> lem is the separation of functional from
> organic disease in the elderly specifically,
> the efficiency of psychological testing as
> a diagnostic tool is even less certain.

Wells goes on to specify the various difficulties. They include dependency of such tests on the willingness and ability of the patient to cooperate, the lack of age norms for many of these tests in the elderly ranges, the overlap in test errors between patients with neruological and functional disorders, and the failure of empirical research (e.g., Matthews, Shaw & Klove, 1966) to demonstrate that neuropsychological tests can reliably discriminate between patients with neurological and functional disorders. Typically, many false positives are found in such research, and so Wells concludes that neuropsychological testing may be quite helpful in ruling out brain damage, but less helpful in ruling it in. In the latter case, there is too great a tendency to call patients with functional disorders brain damaged.

Wells' (1980) critique is actually part of a broader problem having to do with neuropsychological assessment of various forms of presenile and senile dementia, normal aging and cognitive impairment in elderly people with functional psychiatric disorders. Thus, while the standard neuropsychological tests may have difficulties in regard to differentiating between actual dementia and pseudodementia, there are associated difficulties in regard to discriminating between dementia and normal aging, and among the various subtypes of dementia, notably Alzheimer's disease and multi-infarct dementia. With regard to the specific matter of pseudodementia, some neuroscientists might suggest that there may be some difficulty with Wells' conceptualization of the matter. The term "dementia syndrome of depression" has been invented in this regard, to suggest that the condition is not merely an imitation of dementia, but may be a type of real, albeit reversible, dementia. Folstein and McHugh (1978) have suggested that the condition may be produced by some interaction between biochemical alterations associated with depression and the various sources of neuronal depletion associated with aging.

Cohen and Dunner (1980) have pointed out that neuropsychological assessment of elderly individuals with dementia serves the purpose of assisting in diagnosis as well as of providing a knowledge base regarding the nature and rate of cognitive decline. This knowledge base can be used to good advantage in planning for treatment, management and rehabilitation. Reviews of what is known about cognitive decline in dementia have been published in numerous places (Boller et al., this volume, Perez, 1980; Miller, 1981) and will not be repeated here. The important point is that much is known and much more needs to be known about such cognitive processes as memory, language, conceptual abilities and visual-spatial skills in the elderly individual, particularly the elderly individual with dementia.

Neuropsychological assessment of elderly individuals should have particular characteristics and aims. With regard to the matter of characteristics, the use of the standard, relatively lengthy assessment batteries such as the Halstead-Reitan and Luria-Nebrasks batteries has come under question. The demands placed on elderly people by these procedures in regard to such matters as fatigue, complexity and maintenance of attention have raised ethical and scientific questions. Furthermore, the brief "dementia scales" such as the Mini-Mental Status Examination (Folstein, Folstein, & McHugh, 1975), and the Dementia Scale of Blessed, Tomlinson and Roth (1968), have proven to be very effective diagnostic instruments. While these brief structured mental status examinations do not provide detailed information about cognitive function, they do assess degree of dementia, to the extent that Blessed, Tomlinson and Roth (1968) found a +.77 (p < .001) correlation between mean plaque count estimated after death and dementia scores obtained from patients when they were alive. Impressive findings of this type suggest that it is not necessary to administer a full neuropsychological battery if the diagnostic question is simply that of determining presence or absence of dementia, or of estimating its severity. Aside from brevity, another desirable characteristic of neuropsychological tests for the elderly is repeatability, since repeatable instruments can be very useful for tracing the course of dementing illnesses over time.

Most clinicians would probably agree that a major aim of assessment in the elderly is that of distinguishing between treatable and untreatable conditions. This problem area contains two major components, the first of them being diagnostic in nature. Here, the question is often whether or not the patient has a treatable dementia such as normal pressure hydrocephalus or metabolic dementia, dementia syndrome of depression, which is also generally treatable, or one of the irreversible dementias such as Alzheimer's disease. The second component is descriptive in nature and has to do with delineation of cognitive profiles in individual patients. This kind of assessment is particularly useful when active retraining is contemplated such as memory training or language therapy. In this case, the dementia scales are not particularly useful, since one has to know a great deal about the specifics of the patient's memory, language function, psychomotor function, visual-spatial abilities, and related matters. Recent studies in cognitive rehabilitation (Golden, 1978; Diller & Gordon, 1981) have shown how neuropsychological assessment is invaluable in the planning and evaluation of such treatment.

The study of dementia as a neuropsychiatric syndrome is strongly associated with research involving changes in cognitive function associated with the normal aging process. Numerous neuropsychological studies of normal aging have been conducted and there has been a great deal of theoretical exploration of the matter (Klisz, 1978; Kinsbourne, 1980). Various attempts have been made to describe the nature of cognitive changes with age, some emphasizing the significance of psychomotor slowing and others such concepts as crystallized vs. fluid intelligence (Horn & Cattell, 1967), selective deterioration of the right hemisphere (Klisz, 1978; Goldstein & Shelly, 1981), brain age (Reitan, 1973) and selective attention (Kinsbourne, 1980).

There has been extensive investigation of the view that normal aging is like progressive, diffuse brain damage (Goldstein & Shelly, 1975) or like the impairment of neuropsychological function seen in chronic alcoholics (Ryan & Butters, 1980). Perhaps the one conclusion that can be reached from all of these considerations is that whatever changes take place with advancing age are patterned, and do not consist of global intellectual deterioration. This patterning probably has a characteristic temporal course, but there have not been extensive neuropsychologically oriented longitudinal studies capable of documenting this course with any certainty. Furthermore, there has been some suggestion that age related changes are not uniformly progressive, but accelerate markedly shortly before time of death. Riegel and Riegel (1972) have postulated that decline in intellectual function is only seen in individuals who are in the process of dying. Fully healthy individuals, although elderly, do not show intellectual decline.

With regard to the matter of neuropsychological assessment, recent research may be viewed as providing a number of clinically relevant suggestions. First of all, the presence of significant intellectual deficit in an elderly individual in the absence of a history of major systemic illness may reflect the presence of a diagnosable dementia and not merely the effects of normal aging. If a dementia is suspected, there should be further evaluation to determine whether it is of the treatable type. While reversibility of dementia in the elderly is relatively rare, it sometimes occurs. Symptoms of intellectual impairment or frank dementia are frequently seen in elderly depressed individuals, but are rarely seen in younger people with depression. While there is some controversy with regard to whehter this condition is a pseudodementia or an actual dementia, there seems little question that it is treatable as a depression. Following treatment, the intellectual impairment may diminish significantly or essentially disappear. From a practical standpoint, unless neuropsychologically oriented rehabilitation is contemplated making it necessary to acquire detailed information, the brief structured mental status examinations or "dementia scales" are quite satisfactory in regard to establishing the existence of dementia, and may be more practical, feasible and humane to use than the extensive neuropsychological test batteries.

The Neuropsychology of Alcoholism. There is about a twenty year history of systematic neuropsychological research into the effects of chronic alcoholism, utilizing standard tests and test batteries. This research has suggested that alcoholism, aside from being a habit, medical and psychiatric disorder, is a cognitive disorder as well. While alcoholic dementia and deterioration have been observed since antiquity, and the Wernicke-Korsakoff syndrome was noted at least since the late nineteenth century (Wernicke, 1881), subtle adaptive deficits in chronic alcoholics have only been objectively demonstrated during recent years. The pattern of relatively

well preserved language abilities accompanied by substantially impaired complex visual-spatial and conceptual abilities seems quite
well established (Parsons & Farr, 1981). The failure of alcoholics
to perform well on such procedures as the Halstead Category and Wisconsin Card Sorting tests has been observed in many laboratories and
clinics. It now seems apparent that these cognitive deficits found
in large numbers of chronic alcoholics should have strong implications for treatment planning. The significance of these findings
increases when one considers the large and apparently increasing
numbers of chronic alcoholic patients treated in psychiatric facilities. Primary alcoholism in combination with some other mental
disorder accounts for a substantial proportion of populations found
in inpatient and outpatient psychiatric facilities.

The nature of neuropsychological deficit in chronic alcoholics
has been summarized in numerous articles (Goldstein, 1976; Tarter,
1976; Parsons & Farr, 1981). In essence, these reviews have clearly
suggested that alcoholism, if sufficiently severe and chronic, may
be associated with a variety of perceptual and cognitive deficits
that strongly suggest some form of brain dysfunction. It is now a
matter of further delineation of the nature of this dysfunction with
the aim of gaining further understanding of the underlying neuropathology and the connections between this pathology and behavior.
One group of investigators (e.g., Goldstein & Shelly, 1982) have
looked at complex cognitive abilities such as abstraction and visual-
spatial skills utilizing extensive test batteries, while other studies have concentrated on individual skills, notably memory, utilizing
information processing approaches (e.g., Butters & Cermak, 1980a).
These latter investigations have mainly involved patients with alcoholic Korsakoff's syndrome, but chronic alcoholics have also been
studied in this manner (Ryan & Butters, 1980).

Having established the presence of these cognitive deficits in
alcoholics, investigators are now beginning to look at their underlying mechanisms. It seems clear that a long term history of excessive use of alcohol, malnutrition, possible multiple head trauma and
alcoholism related systemic illnesses is likely to eventuate in some
degree of impaired brain function. The questions that now arise have
to do with a variety of matters having to do with the nature of this
dysfunction. One major question has to do with recoverability following abstinence and restoration of good nutrition. Other questions
involve underlying brain mechanisms both with regard to localization
of the brain damage in various alcoholism related syndromes (Goldstein & Shelly, 1982) and the nature of the neuropathology.
Still, other questions have to do with individual differences, with
a strong emphasis on genetic factors. There is some evidence for
a genetic predisposition for alcoholism in general, and there may
also be genetic, as well as sex, differences in susceptibility to
brain pathology, as well as pathology of other organs and organ
systems among alcoholic individuals. Tarter (1976) has suggested

that early life minimal brain damage and/or hyperkinesis may be a predisposing factor for the acquisition of alcoholism. Investigators have looked at similarities between alcoholism and other diseases, as well as between alcoholism and aging. For example, there are certain similarities and possible continuties among Korsakoff's syndrome, chronic alcoholism and Alzheimer's disease (Ryan & Butters, 1980; Butters, 1982). Parsons and Farr (1981), after conducting a review of the pertinent studies, concluded that the pattern of neuropsychological deficit commonly found among chronic alcoholics is not essentially different from what is found among patients with a variety of organic brain diseases.

The literature on neuropsychological assessment of alcoholics has been based largely on the Halstead-Reitan battery, including the Wechsler scales, and a relatively small number of other tests; notably the Wisconsin Card Sorting test and the Witkin Rod and Frame test. Recently, however, Chmielewski and Golden (1980), have demonstrated that the Luria-Nebraska Neuropsychological battery is also sensitive to the effects of alcoholism. In all cases, alcoholics tended to perform poorly on tests of complex cognitive abilities and relatively well on tests of simpler skills. As suggested above, while it may be difficult to discriminate among alcoholics and patients with a number of organic brain diseases through the use of neuropsychological test batteries, it is likely that some degree of deficit will be seen among members of many alcoholic populations. While the degree of deficit may vary with such factors as age, education and socio-economic status, in general, the chronic alcoholic patient is quite likely to demonstrate deficit relative to a non-alcoholic who is matched along these dimensions. This proposition is well supported in a study by Ryan and Butters (1980) in which such careful matching was accomplished. Here, the alcoholic subjects did substantially worse on a series of memory tasks than their well matched controls.

There is some evidence that alcoholism accelerates the aging process (Jones & Parsons, 1972). Therefore, assessment of elderly patients with alcoholic histories may reveal substantial deficits at a far more severe level than would be found for normal elderly individuals. We have found that in these cases it is often difficult to tell whether the patient has alcoholism, Alzheimer's disease or a combination of the two. Further research is clearly needed in this area with the aim of possible elicitation of different performance patterns between the two disorders. The matter is of some importance because the prognoses for the two disorders are quite different from each other. In the case of alcoholism, there may be no substantial progression as long as the patient remains abstinent and well nourished, while progressive deterioration can be expected in the case of Alzheimer's disease regardless of the patient's dietary and related habits.

It should go without saying that neuropsychological assessment
of alcoholic patients is generally not for the purpose of determining whether the patient is an alcoholic or not; something that can
be determined far more directly. Rather, assessment of alcoholics
generally is accomplished for purposes of assessing amount and pattern of disability, while longitudinal assessment may be accomplished
to estimate degree of recovery. With regard to the latter matter,
several of the reviews of the recovery literature (Goodwin & Hill,
1975; Tarter, 1976; Parsons & Farr, 1981) indicate that there is
some recovery of cognitive abilities in alcoholics following a period
of abstinence. However, there is substantial evidence that certain
functions recover but others do not. For example, Goldman and Rosenbaum (1977) found recovery on a verbal, but not a visual paired-associate, task. Ryan, DiDario, Butters and Adinolfi (1980) report that
while alcoholics may show some recovery on digit substitution and
some attention tests, they remain impaired following a year of abstinence on tests of learning and memory. Thus, while the neuropsychologist might expect to find some modest degree of recovery in
cognitive abilities, it now seems apparent that certain abilities
become permanently impaired in chronic alcoholics. Grant, Reed and
Adams (1980) have attempted to place this research into a conceptual
model for the natural history of alcohol and drug-related disorders,
stressing the necessity of developing methodologies for understanding
alcohol-neuropsychological relationships.

The assessment of amount and pattern of disability would appear
to have particular implications for remediation. Perhaps the most
straightforward illustration of this point is in the area of memory
and memory training. In order to effectively implement such training in amnesic alcoholics, it would seem crucial to understand the
nature of their memory deficits. For example, Cermak (1977) has been
able to improve memory in Korsakoff patients using methods based on
what was known about the nature of the memory disorder in this condition. Binder and Schreiber (1980) have done similar work. It is
quite likely that the same methods would not work with patients having different types of amnesia. Similarly, Goldstein, Chotlos,
McCarthy and Neuringer (1968), aware of the gait difficulties commonly found among chronic but sober alcoholics, were able to accom-
plish effective gait training. It is also felt, but only demonstrated in a few studies (e.g., Gregson & Taylor, 1977), that there
is a relationship between neuropsychological test performance and
such important clinical factors as treatment outcome and social com-
petence.

The clinician doing detailed assessments of alcoholic patients
might wish to have the capability of discriminating among certain
subtypes of the disorder. The major distinction appears to be between chronic alcoholism and alcoholic amnestic (Korsakoff's) syndrome. From the point of view of neuropsychological assessment, it
is necessary to do formal memory testing with some instrument like

the Wechsler Memory Scale in order to diagnose Korsakoff's syndrome. The MQ or other index of memory ability should be substantially lower than the IQ, which should be in the average range. While chronic alcoholics can also be expected to have average level IQs, they should not show a very wide discrepancy between IQ and MQ. Butters and Cermak (1980) found a 20-30 point discrepancy between IQ and MQ with their Korsakoff patients. The other important matter to consider is antecedent neuropsychological deficit. In some cases, apparent alcoholism related deficit may not in fact be alcoholism related but may instead reflect the consequences of a developmental disorder. In effect, some alcoholics may perform in the impaired ranges of certain neuropsychological tests not because of the alcoholism but because of some antedating deficiency in cognitive development. It is often quite difficult to determine whether failure on some test is the result of an adult acquired disability or of the fact that the test measures an ability at which the patient never did well. Investigators such as Tarter (1976) have examined this matter through the use of a checklist, given to the parent if possible, containing a list of manifestations of early life neurological dysfunction, such as hyperactivity. Clinically, it would seem to be quite important to know whether observed deficits are adult acquired or developmental phenomena.

SUMMARY

A brief survey was conducted of neuropsychological assessment of patients having five classes of psychiatric disorder: schizophrenia, temporal lobe disorders, affective disorders, dementia of the presenile and senile period, and alcoholism. While assessment of such patients deviates somewhat from the traditional focus of clinical neuropsychology on structural brain disease, recent research has strongly suggested that each of the above conditions have significant neuropsychological implications. Furthermore, many clinical neuropsychologists continue to be faced with the traditional problems of discriminating between the so-called functional and organic mental disorders. This latter problem may be in the process of being substantially resolved through extensive neurobehavioral research into the psychiatric disorders. This research has tended to encourage a reformulation of the diagnostic questions as they were originally asked, since the assumption that certain functional disorders do not have a neurological basis is being called into question. This situation seems to be particularly pertinent in the case of schizophrenia, since direct evidence of abnormal brain structure and function continues to be found; primarily through the application of advanced brain imaging techniques. Thus, it now seems quite appropriate to look at the neuropsychological aspects of these syndromes, not so much to determine whether the patient has a "functional" or "organic" disorder, but more to formulate observed behavior of these patients in information processing or brain-behavior relationship terms. Here, we have attempted to

briefly describe some of the research findings and remaining problems
in neuropsychological assessment of individuals with these disorders.

REFERENCES

Adams, K.M. In search of Luria's battery: A false start. Journal
    of Consulting and Clinical Psychology, 1980, 48, 511-516.
Bard, P. Emotion I: The neuro-humoral basis of emotional reactions.
    In C. Murchison (Ed.). Handbook of general experimental psych-
    ology. Worcester, MA: Clark University Press, 1934.
Bear, D., & Fedio, P. Quantitative analysis of interictal behavior
    in temporal lobe epilepsy. Archives of Neurology, 1977, 34
    454-467.
Binder, L.M., & Schreiber, V. Visual imagery and verbal mediation
    as memory aids in recovering alcoholics. Journal of Clinical
    Neuropsychology, 1980, 2, 71-73.
Blessed, G., Tomlinson, B.C., & Roth, M. The association between
    quantitative measures of dementia and senile change in the
    cerebral gray matter of elderly subjects. British Journal of
    Psychiatry, 1968, 114, 797-811.
Boll, T.J., Heaton, R., & Reitan, R.M. Neuropsychological and emo-
    tional correlates of Huntington's chorea. The Journal of Ner-
    vous and Mental Disease, 1974, 158, 61-69.
Boller, F., Detre, T., & Kim, Y. Temporal lobes and overlap between
    neurology, psychiatry and neuropsychology. In P.E. Logue & J.
    M. Shear (Eds.). Clinical neuropsychology: A multi-disciplinary
    approach. (In press.)
Bruder, G.E., & Yozawitz, A. Central auditory processing and later-
    alization in psychiatric patients. In J. Gruzelier & P. Flor-
    Henry (Eds.). Hemisphere asymmetries of function in psychopath-
    ology. Amsterdam: Elsevier/North Holland, 1979.
Buchsbaum, M.S. New visions of the brain. Guest Lecture Series,
    Western Psychiatric Institute and Clinic, March 1981. Andrew
    M. Browne Memorial Lecture.
Butters, N. Memory disorders of demented and amnesic patients: A
    comparative approach. In M. Meier (Chm.), Dementia II: Neuro-
    psychological analysis of dementia. Symposium presented at the
    International Neuropsychological Society, Pittsburgh, PA, 1982.
Butters, N., & Cermak, L.W. Alcoholic Korsakoff's Syndrome: An in-
    formation-processing approach to America. New York: Academic
    Press, 1980.
Cannon, W.B. The James-Lange theory of emotion: A critical examina-
    tion and an alternative theory. American Journal of Psychology,
    1927, 106-124.
Cannon, W.B. Bodily changes in pain hunger, fear and rage: An ac-
    count of recent researches into the function of emotional ex-
    citement. New York: Appleton, 1929.
Cermak, L.S. Improving retention in alcoholic Korsakoff patients.
    In O.A. Parsons (Chm), Behavioral assessment of cognitive

functioning in alcoholics: Treatment implications. Symposium presented at the NATO International Conference on Experimental and Behavioral Approaches to Alcoholism, Bergen, Norway, 1977.

Chmielewski, C., & Golden, C.J.   Alcoholism and brain damage: An investigation using the Luria-Nebraska Neuropsychological Battery. Journal of Neuroscience, 1980, 10, 99-105.

Cohen, D., & Dunner, D.   The assessment of cognitive dysfunction in dementing illness.   In J.O. Cole & J.E. Barrett (Eds.), Psychopathology in the aged.   New York: Raven Press, 1980.

D'Elia, G., & Perris, C.   Cerebral functional dominance and depression: An analysis of EEG amplitude in depressed patients.   Acta Psychiatrica Scandinavia, 1974, 49, 191-197.

Diller, L., & Gordon, W.A.   Rehabilitation and clinical neuropsychology.   In S.B. Filskov & T.J. Boll (Eds.), Handbook of clinical neuropsychology.   New York: Wiley-Interscience, 1981.

Dikmen, S., & Reitan, R.M.   MMPI correlates of dysphasic language disturbances.   Journal of Abnormal Psychology, 1974, 83, 675-679.

Flor-Henry, P., & Yeudall, L.T.   Neuropsychological investigation of schizophrenia and manic-depressive psychoses.   In J. Gruzelier & P. Flor-Henry (Eds.), Hemisphere asymmetries of function in psychopathology.   Amsterdam: Elsevier/North Holland, 1979.

Folstein, M.F., Folstein, S.E., & McHugh, P.R.   "Mini-mental State:" A practical method for grading the cognitive state of patients for the clinician.   Journal of Psychiatric Research, 1975, 12, 189-198.

Friedman, A.S.   Minimal effects of severe depression in cognitive functioning.   Journal of Abnormal and Social Psychology, 1964, 69, 237-243.

Gainotti, G.   Emotional behavior and hemispheric side of the lesion. Cortex, 1972, 8, 41-55.

Golden, C.J.   Diagnosis and rehabilitation in clinical neuropsychology.   Springfield, IL: C.C. Thomas, 1978.

Golden, C.J., Moses, J.A., Zelazowski, R., Graber, G., Zatz, L.M., Horvath, T.B., & Berger, P.A.   Cerebral ventricular size and neuropsychological impairment in young chronic schizophrenics. Archives of General Psychiatry, 1980, 37, 619-623.

Goldman, M.S., & Rosenbaum, G.   Psychological recoverability following chronic alcohol abuse.   In F. Seixas (Ed.), Currents in alcoholism, Vol. 2.   New York: Grune & Stratton, 1977.

Goldstein, G.   Perceptual and cognitive deficit in alcoholics.   In G. Goldstein & C. Neuringer (Eds.), Empirical studies of alcoholism.   Cambridge, MA: Ballinger, 1976.

Goldstein, G.   Cognitive and perceptual differences between schizophrenics and organics.   Schizophrenia Bulletin, 1978, 4, 160-195.

Goldstein, G., Chotlos, J.W., McCarthy, R.J., & Neuringer, C.   Recovery from gait instability in alcoholics.   Quarterly Journal of Studies on Alcohol, 1968, 29, 38-43.

Goldstein, G., & Halperin, K.M. Neuropsychological differences among subtypes of schizophrenia. Journal of Abnormal Psychology, 1977, 86, 36-40.

Goldstein, G., & Scheerer, M. Abstract and concrete behavior: An experimental study with special tests. Psychological Monographs, 1941, 53, (2, Whole No. 239).

Goldstein, G., & Shelly, C.H. Similarities and differences between psychological deficit in aging and brain damage. Journal of Gerontology, 1975, 30, 448-455.

Goldstein, G., & Shelly, C.H. Does the right hemisphere age more rapidly than the left? Journal of Clinical Neuropsychology, 1981, 3, 65-78.

Goldstein, G., & Shelly, C. A multivariate neuropsychological approach to brain lesion localization in alcoholism. Addictive Behaviors, 1982, 7, 165-175.

Goldstein, S.G., Filskov, S.B., Weaver, L.A., & Ives, J.A. Neuropsychological effects of electroconvulsive therapy. Journal of Clinical Psychology, 1977, 33, 798-806.

Goodwin, D.W., & Hill, S.Y. Chronic effects of alcohol and other psychoactive drugs on intellect, learning and memory. In J. Rankin (Ed.). Alcohol, drugs, and brain damage. Ontario: Addiction Research Foundation, 1975.

Gordon, H., Goldstein, G., & Sabol, W. Hemispheric asymmetries in chronic schizophrenia. Paper presented at a meeting of the International Neuropsychological Society, Pittsburgh, PA, 1982.

Grant, I., Reed, R., & Adams, K. Natural history of alcohol and drug-related brain disorder: Implications for neuropsychological research. Journal of Clinical Neuropsychology, 1980, 2, 321-331.

Gregson, R.A.M., & Taylor, G.M. Prediction of relapse in men alcoholics. Journal of Studies on Alcohol, 1977, 38, 1749-1759.

Gruzelier, J. Lateral asymmetries in electodermal activity and psychosis. In J. Gruzelier & P. Flor-Henry (Eds.). Hemisphere asymmetries of function in psychopathology. Amsterdam: Elsevier/North Holland, 1979.

Gruzelier, J., & Flor-Henry, P. (Eds.) Hemisphere asymmetries of function in psychopathology. Amsterdam: Elsevier/North Holland, 1979.

Gur, R.E. Left hemispheric dysfunction and left hemispheric overactivation in schizophrenia. Journal of Abnormal Psychology, 1978, 87, 226-238.

Heaton, R.K., Baade, L.E., & Johnson, K.L. Neuropsychological test results associated with psychiatric disorders in adults. Psychological Bulletin, 1978, 85, 141-162.

Heaton, R.K., & Crowley, T.J. Effects of psychiatric disorders and their somatic treatments on neuropsychological test results. In S.B. Filskov & T.J. Boll (Eds.), Handbook of clinical neuropsychology. New York: Wiley-Interscience, 1981.

Horn, J.L., & Cattell, R.B. Age differences in fluid and crystallized intelligence. Acta Psychologica, 1967, 26, 107-129.

Ingvar, D.H., Brun, A., Hagberg, B., & Gustafson, L. Regional cerebral blood flow in the dominant hemisphere in confirmed cases
of Alzheimer's disease, Pick's disease, and multi-infarct dementia: Relationship to clinical symptomatology and neuropathological findings. In R. Katzman, R.D. Terry, & K.L. Bick (Eds.),
Alzheimer's disease: Senile dementia and related disorders. New
York: Raven Press, 1978.

James, W. The principles of psychology. New York: Holt, 1980.

Jones, B.M., & Parsons, O.A. Specific vs. generalized deficits of
abstracting ability in chronic alcoholics. Archives of General
Psychiatry, 1972, 26, 380-384.

Kietzman, M.L., Sutton, S., & Zubin, J. Experimental approaches to
psychopathology. New York: Academic Press, 1975.

Kinsbourne, M. Attentional dysfunctions and the elderly: Theoretical models and research perspectives. In L.W. Poon, J.L.
Fozard, L.S. Cermak, D. Arenberg, & L.W. Thompson (Eds.), New
directions in memory and aging. Hillsdale, NJ: Lawrence Erlbaum
Associates, 1980.

Klisz, D. Neuropsychological evaluation in older persons. In M.
Storandt, I.C. Siegler, & M.F. Elias (Eds.). The clinical psychology of aging. New York: Plenum Press, 1978.

Klove, H., & Matthews, C.G. Neuropsychological studies of patients
with epilepsy. In R.M. Reitan & L.A. Davison (Eds.), Clinical
neuropsychology: Current status and application. New York:
Winston-Wiley, 1974.

Kral, V.A. Benign senescent forgetfulness. In R. Katzman, R.D.
Terry, & K.L. Bick (Eds.), Alzheimer's disease: Senile dementia
and related disorders. New York: Raven Press, 1978.

Kronfol, A., Hamsher, K., Digre, K., & Waziri, R. Depression and
hemispheric functions: Changes associated with unilateral ECT.
British Journal of Psychiatry, 1978, 132, 560-567.

Levit, A.L., Sutton, S., & Zubin, J. Evoked potential correlates
of information processing in psychiatric patients. Psychological Medicine, 1973, 3, 487-494.

Luchins, D.J., Weinberger, D.R., & Wyatt, R.J. Schizophrenia: Evidence of a subgroup with reversed cerebral asymmetry. Archives
of General Psychiatry, 1979, 36, 1309-1311.

Magaro, P.A. Information processing and hemispheric specialization
in schizophrenia and paranoia. Paper presented at American
Psychological Association meeting, Toronto, Canada, 1978.

Malec, J. Neuropsychological assessment of schizophrenia vs. brain
damage: A review. Journal of Nervous and Mental Disease, 1978,
166, 507-516.

Matthews, C.G., Cleeland, S.C., & Hopper, C.L. Neuropsychological
patterns in multiple sclerosis. Diseases of the Nervous System, 1970, 31, 161-170.

Matthews, C.G., Shaw, D.J., & Klove, H. Psychological test performances in neurologic and "pseudoneurologic" subjects. Cortex,
1966, 2, 244-253.

Mettler, F.A. (Ed.) Selective partial ablation of the frontal cortex. New York: Hoeber, 1949.

Miller, E. The nature of the cognitive decline in dementia. In N.E. Miller & G.D. Cohen (Eds.). Clinical aspects of Alzheimer's disease and senile dementia. New York: Raven Press, 1981.

Miller, N.E., & Cohen, G.D. Clinical aspects of Alzheimer's disease and dementia. New York: Raven Press, 1981.

Perez, F.I. Behavioral studies of dementia: Methods of investigation and analysis. In J.O. Cole & J.E. Barrett (Eds.). Psychopathology of the aged. New York: Raven Press, 1980.

Perkins, C.W. Some correlates of Category Test scores for nonorganic psychiatric patients. Journal of Clinical Psychology, 1974, 30, 176-178.

Perris, C., & Monakhov, K. Depressive symptomatology and systemic structural analysis of the EEG. In J. Gruzelier & P. Flor-Henry (Eds.). Hemisphere asymmetries of function in psychopathology. Amsterdam: Elsevier/North Holland, 1979.

Parsons, O.A., & Farr, S.P. The neuropsychology of alcohol and drug use. In S.B. Filskov & T.J. Boll (Eds.). Handbook of clinical neuropsychology. New York: Wiley-Interscience, 1981.

Purisch, A.D., Golden, C.J., & Hammeke, T.A. Discrimination of schizophrenic and brain-injured patients by a standardized version of Luria's neuropsychological tests. Journal of Consulting and Clinical Psychology, 1978, 46, 1266-1273.

Rapaport, D., Gill, M., & Schafer, R. Diagnostic psychological testing. Chicago, IL: Year Book Publishers, 1945.

Rieder, R.O., Donnelly, E.G., Herdt, J.R., & Waldman, I.N. Sulcal prominence in young chronic schizophrenic patients: CT scan findings associated with impairment on neuropsychological tests. Psychiatry Research, 1979, 1, 1-8.

Riegel, K.F., & Riegel, R.M. Development, drugs and death. Develmental Psychology, 1972, 6, 302-319.

Reitan, R.M. Behavioral manifestations of impaired brain functions in aging. Paper presented at a meeting of the American Psychological Association, Montreal, 1973.

Rosenthal, R., & Bigelow, L.B. Quantitative brain measures in chronic schizophrenia. British Journal of Psychiatry, 1972, 121, 259-264.

Ryan, C., & Butters, N. Further evidence for a continuum-of-impairment encompassing male alcoholic Korsakoff patients and chronic alcoholic men. Alcoholism: Clinical and Experimental Research, 1980, 4, 190-198.

Ryan, C., DiDario, B., Butters, N., & Adinolfi, A. The relationship between abstinence and recovery of function in male alcoholics. Journal of Clinical Neuropsychology, 1980, 2, 125-134.

Squire, L.R., Slater, P.C., & Chace, P.M. Retrograde amnesia: Temporal gradient in very long term memory following electroconvulsive therapy. Science, 1975, 187, 77-79.

Stevens, J.R. Psychiatric implications of psychomotor epilepsy. Archives of General Psychiatry, 1966, 14, 461-471.

Tarter, R. Neuropsychological investigation of alcoholism. In G.

Goldstein & C. Neuringer (Eds.). Empirical studies of alcoholism. Cambridge, MA: Ballinger, 1976.

Valenstein, E., & Heilman, K.M. Emotional disorders resulting from lesions of the central nervous system. In K.M. Heilman, & E. Valenstein (Eds.). Clinical neuropsychology. New York: Oxford University Press, 1979.

Walsh, K.W. Neuropsychology: A clinical approach. Edinburgh: Churchill Livingston, 1978.

Watson, C.G., Davis, W.E., & Gasser, B. The separation of organics from depressives with ability-personality-based tests. Journal of Clinical Psychology, 1978, 34, 393-397.

Wells, C.E. The differential diagnosis of psychiatric disorders in the elderly. In J.O. Cole & J.E. Barrett (Eds.). Psychopathology in the aged. New York: Raven Press, 1980.

Wernicke, C. Lehrbuch der gehirnkrankeiten fur arzte und sturdierende. Berlin: Fisher, 1881.

Zubin, J., & Steinhauer, S. How to break the logjam in schizophrenia: A look beyond genetics. Journal of Nervous and Mental Disease, 1981, 169, 477-492.

ALZHEIMER AND RELATED DEMENTIAS: A REVIEW OF CURRENT KNOWLEDGE

François Boller,[1] Gerald Goldstein,[2] Carol Dorr,[3]
Youngjai Kim,[1] John Moossy,[4] Eldred Richey,[5]
Diane Wagener,[1] and Sidney K. Wolfson, Jr.[6]

Department of Psychiatry, Western Psychiatric Institute
and Clinic, University of Pittsburgh, Pittsburgh, PA[1];
Highland Drive Veterans Administration Medical Center,
Pittsburgh, PA[2]; Yale New Haven Hospital, New Haven, CT[3];
Presbyterian University Hospital, Pittsburgh, PA[4]; Univer-
sity of Alabama Medical School, Mobile, AL[5]; and Montefiore
Hospital, Pittsburgh, PA[6]

This paper will review some of the information which has recently
become available concerning the neuropsychology, chemistry, physiology
and pathology of Alzheimer Disease (AD) and other related dementias of
aging. Despite the devastating impact of these diseases on society,
they are difficult to diagnose with certainty during life. This diagnostic difficulty has considerably hampered attempts to manage and
treat these diseases. In this paper, we will first review the epidemiology of these conditions and discuss some current hypotheses
concerning their possible etiologies. We will then discuss current
diagnostic considerations with special emphasis on neuropsychology
and conclude with a brief description of the clinical criteria presently used to diagnose AD and the related dementias of aging. It
is hoped that this review of current knowledge will stimulate research aimed at improving the diagnosis and eventual therapy of these
conditions.

Epidemiology of AD and Other Dementias of Aging

Dementia, defined as a deterioration of intellectual functions
due to organic disease of the central nervous system, is estimated
to affect almost two million persons in the United States and, in
about 50% of those cases, it is severe enough to require institutionalization. While it represents a symptom of many disorders (Haase,

1977), only a relatively small number of diseases are known to cause most cases of dementia (Marsden & Harrison, 1972; Corkin, Growdon, Sullivan, & Shedlack, 1981). AD in both its presenile and senile forms accounts for more than 50% of the persons with moderate to severe dementia and, therefore, probably affects over half a million persons in this country. Blumenthal (draft) has suggested that within a four year period, approximately three-quarters of the people with a serious organic brain syndrome can be expected to die; Alzheimer Disease alone is estimated to produce from 60,000 to 90,000 annual deaths in excess of what would be expected based on age (Katzman, 1976).

An additional sizeable percentage of all dementias is caused by multi-infarct dementia (MID) (Hachinski, Lassen, & Marshall, 1974) and other vascular disease (Loizou, Kendall, & Marshall, 1981; Heyman, 1978). The reported prevalence varies from 10% (Marsden & Harrison, 1972) to 30%-40% (Busse & Blazer, 1980). One must recognize, however, that there is currently a steep decrease in the incidence of strokes (Garraway, Whisnant, Furlan, Phillips, Kurland, & O'Fallon, 1979); therefore, this figure may decrease in future studies. Similarly, the number of patients with both AD and vascular changes may be expected to decline.

The issue of "dementia syndrome of depression" or "pseudo-dementia" is more controversial. There is clearly considerable overlap between dementia and depression. Katzman and Karasu (1975) point out that "25% of patients with dementia may be depressed." On the other hand, some degree of cognitive impairment is found in up to 50% of depressed patients (Folstein & McHugh, 1978). The terms "dementia syndrome of depression" or "pseudo-dementia" are reserved, however, for elderly depressives showing a mental status that simulates a dementing process. It has been estimated that this syndrome is found in 15% of elderly persons presenting with dementia (Roth, 1976). The name "pseudo-dementia" is actually misleading and the term "dementia syndrome of depression" is probably preferable because the latter implies that a neuropathological mechanism should be expected in these cases. Epidemiological research suggests that the dementia of depressed patients is highly reversible since comprehensive follow-up studies have shown that "the overlap in long-term outcome between depression and dementia is virtually nil" (Roth, 1978a, 1980b).

Other forms of dementia that are often confused with AD include Creutzfeldt-Jakob Disease (CJD), a condition which is now attributed to a transmissible agent. This disease is certainly rare, since only about 200 cases were said to have been reported until 1977 (Haase, 1977); however, some authors estimate that it is found in about three percent of autopsied dementia cases (Wells, 1978). The real incidence may lie somewhere between those two figures. As suggested by a careful epidemiological study currently in progress in Great Britain, the data so far have indicated an incidence of 0.31/million (Matthews & Will, 1982). Pick's Disease has been said to be as frequent as AD (Sjogren, Sjogren, & Lindgren, 1952) but, for reasons that are unclear, it is not frequently diagnosed neuropathologically in North America. Other conditions, such as subcortical gliosis (Neumann & Cohn, 1967), are certainly even more rare. Finally, a certain number of patients diagnosed clinically as having AD do not show the characteristic Alzheimer changes or neuropathological evidence of other diseases and for these the term "simple senile atrophy" has been recommended (Haase, 1977).

Many other diseases ranging from some that affect primarily the Central Nervous System (CNS) (e.g., Huntington Disease - HD) to some general medical diseases (e.g., hypothyroidism) are responsible for a considerable percentage of dementia cases. They will not be reviewed here because they often occur at an earlier age and/or are usually accompanied by other prominent signs and symptoms of CNS or general medical disorders. These diseases should be easily diagnosed or ruled out early in the assessment of demented patients.

To date, no formal study of the epidemiology of dementia has been carried out in the Pittsburgh area. Table 1 summarizes the pathological diagnoses in 115 autopsy cases collected from 1973 until June 1981 from the files of the Division of Neuropathology of the University of Pittsburgh Medical School. During that period of time, 1664 autopsies including CNS examination had been performed at Presbyterian University Hospital. The diagnoses of AD, Pick and CJD are based on both the classical clinical manifestations and the neuropathological findings. Obviously, this hospital-based sample does not allow one to draw inferences about the prevalence and incidence of dementia in the general population; nevertheless, several interesting observations may be made.

Besides the high percentage of cases with Pick's Disease and CJD, the most striking figure in this series is the high number of cases in which macroscopic atrophy was not accompanied by microscopic findings typical of AD or other specific conditions. On the other hand, the percentage of subjects with lacunar infarcts is relatively high. Furthermore, it could not be determined how many patients with lacunar infarctions were actually demented.

Etiology and Pathogenesis of Dementia in the Aged

Alzheimer disease. There are some indications that presenile dementia (with onset before age 65) and senile dementia (onset age 65 and over) may differ in some respects. A relatively recent review of the problem (Katzman, Terry, & Bick, 1978b) has pointed out that this distinction may help uncover different, but yet unknown, etiological factors. Regardless of the age of onset, however, the

Table 1. Alzheimer Disease and other dementias: Pathological
          diagnoses in 115 cases drawn from the autopsy population
          of Presbyterian-University Hospital and outside consul-
          tations, January 1, 1973 to June 30, 1981.

	N	%
Alzheimer Disease	17	15
Pick's Disease	4	3.5
Creutzfeldt-Jakob Disease	6	5
Huntington's Disease	4	3.5
Progressive Supranuclear Palsy	1	1
NFT: SP: GVD (1)	8	7
"Cortical Atrophy: (2)	20	17
Lacunar Infarctions (3)	55	48
Total	115	100

(1) Microscopic examination revealed neurofibrillary tangles (NFT);
    Senile plaques (SP); Granular vacuolar degeneration (GVD).

(2) Despite the gross impression of diffuse cerebral atrophy ranging
    from mild to severe, microscopic examination did not demonstrate
    NFT or SP or GVD and clinical evidence of dementia as recorded in
    the hospital charts was inclusive, incomplete or inadequate.

(3) Three or more old cavitary infarcts 0.2-1.5 cm. in 2 or more of
    the following sites: corpus striatum and/or internal capsule;
    thalamus; pontine base; cerebellar white matter; central cere-
    bral white matter.

neuropathological changes of AD are not very specific, as shown by
their occurrence in many conditions other than AD (Mortimer, 1980).
It is, therefore, possible that AD may represent a final common
neuropathological pathway for many different diseases. Nevertheless,
for the purpose of this review, we will follow the common practice
(Mortimer & Schuman, 1981), of viewing AD as a unitary process, and
will consider both the presenile and senile forms. We will only
distinguish one form from the other when the separation appears to
be valid.

    Although the etiology and pathogenesis of AD remain unknown,
we shall briefly review some of the hypotheses that are currently
being entertained.

    Genetic hypothesis. The possibility that genetic factors may
play a role in the etiology of AD is indicated by the increased risk
of dementia in relatives of AD patients. Larsson, Sjogren and Jacob-

son (1952) found an increased risk of senile dementia in first degree relatives of Alzheimer probands. In a series of studies conducted on families from Minnesota (Heston, 1977, 1978), the increased risk for secondary cases of AD in relatives was again demonstrated. In this same sampling of families, Heston and his collaborators (Heston & Mastri, 1977; Heston, 1979) also noted increased risk of Down's Syndrome, lymphoproliferative cancers, autoimmune disorders and other immune function related problems. In general, a greater risk has been demonstrated for relatives of presenile dementia probands than for relatives of senile dementia probands.

It is also clear that genetic factors or vulnerability alone cannot explain the occurrence of AD. In two studies, monozygotic twins were reported who were discordant for AD (Davidson & Roberson, 1965; Hunter, Dayan, & Wilson, 1972). Discordant monozygotic twins do not disprove a single genetic vulnerability, since genetically vulnerable individuals may or may not manifest a disease (penetrance) because of other environmental stresses. The observation that the incidence of AD is significantly greater in women than in men (Aakesson, 1969), is another indication that environment has a role in the expression of the disease. This increase in occurrence in females is not simply due to the earlier mortality of males.

The nature of any specific genetic factor has not been demonstrated, but certain associations have been noted. Heston (1977) speculated that the primary common lesion in AD and the other disorders clustered in the families he studied involves microtubules. He noted that, "tubules and filamentous organelles are integrally involved in immune phenomena" (Heston, 1978). These microfilamentous structures are also responsible for pulling chromosomes away from the equator of the cell during division. If there is abnormal microtubular physiology, nondisjunctions would presumably occur more frequently than expected. This would explain the increased frequency of Down's Syndrome in these families. In addition, the proteins from the tubules found in the Alzheimer brain have abnormal solubilities (Nishimura, Harigrichi, & Tada, 1975).

The frequent occurrence of AD in patients with Down's Syndrome who survive beyond age 30 years has stimulated cytogenetic studies and one report (Ward, Cook, Robinson, & Austin, 1979) has claimed significant increases of aneuploidy in both sporadic and familial AD. A later paper (White, Crandall, Goudsmit, Morrow, Alling, Gajdusek, & Tijio, 1981) has failed to confirm this finding: no increase in aneuploidy or aberrations was formed in either AD patients or their relatives.

In conclusion, the precise role of genetic factors in AD remains uncertain, perhaps because of the complexity and cost of thorough epidemiologic studies. It does appear, however, to be one of the most important areas for future research.

Immunological hypothesis. Both clinical and experimental data
suggest that immunological factors may play a crucial role in AD.
It has been noted for several years that aging is accompanied by a
decrease in function of the immune system which appears to parallel
the rise in the incidence of AD (Walford, 1967). Brain-specific
antibodies (gammaglobulins) increase in the serum with aging in both
experimental animals and humans; furthermore, some AD patients have
significantly higher levels of such antibodies than age-matched controls (Nandy, 1978). Ishii and Haga (1976) have demonstrated the
presence of fragments of immunoglobulins in senile plaques (SP). A
link between immunological and genetic factors may be provided by
the findings of Stem and Op Den Veld (1978) concerning an increase
in HP1 (one of two allelic genes that are thought to control human
serum haptoglobins) in the presenile form of AD (which they call
Alzheimer-Fischer Disease). The precise significance of these immunological findings, like many other findings related to the various hypotheses concerning the etiology of dementia, remains unde-
termined.

Neurochemical hypothesis. The demonstration a few years ago
that a specific neurochemical deficit is consistently present in AD
(Davies & Maloney, 1976; Bowen, Smith, White, & Davidson, 1976;
Perry, Gibson, Blessed, Perry, & Tomlinson, 1977a; Perry, Perry,
Blessed, & Tomlinson, 1977b; White, Hiley, & Goodhardt, 1977), probably represents the most important recent advance in our understanding of the disease. It has been shown that brains of AD patients
have, in over 50% of cases, a reduced activity in some of the enzymes
involved in acetylcholine (ACh) metabolism, particularly choline ace-
tyltransferase (CAT) and acetylcholinesterase. This decrease has
been shown to correlate with both neuropathological (Perry, Perry,
Blessed, & Tomlinson, 1977b) and cognitive (Perry, Tomlinson, Bergmann, Gibson, & Perry, 1978) changes in AD. There is evidence that
the presynaptic part of the cholinergic system is selectively involved in the disease. The catecholamine system, however, may also
be abnormal in AD as inferred from a decline in homovanilic acid and
5 hydroxyindalacetic acid in the cerebrospinal fluid (CSF) of patients with AD, especiálly those with the presenile form (Gottfries,
Gottfries, & Ross, 1969a,b). Cells belonging to the gamma-amino-
butyric acid (GABA) system are also affected (Reisine, Yamamaura,
Bird, Spokes, & Enna, 1978). There are reasons to believe that the
abnormal ACh enzymes are due to a relative loss of cholinergic neurons with only a relative sparing of adrenergic neurons.

Several attempts have recently been made to improve the dementia
of AD by raising plasma choline levels, or by using anticholines-
terase-like drugs. The often mixed results of these therapeutic
trials may be due to the fact that the catecholamine and GABA systems
are also affected in addition to the ACh system. However, even if
no valid treatment of dementia has yet emerged from these neurochemical studies, they have already made crucial contributions to our

understanding of the pathogenesis of AD and they may in the future provide the most reliable diagnostic marker of the disease.

Exogenous hypothesis. A few years ago, Crapper and collaborators (Crapper, Krishman, & Dalton, 1973; Crapper, Krishman, & Quittkat, 1976) reported an increased concentration of aluminum (Al) in the brains of AD patients and suggested, on the basis of previous animal work, that neurofibrillary tangles (NFT) (one of the intracellular neuropathological changes found in AD), are in part due to Al intoxication. More recently there has been evidence militating against Al playing a major role in the disease. One study conducted (McDermott, Smith, & Iqbal, 1977) did not find differences in Al concentrations between AD and age-matched controls. Also the "NFT" induced in rats by experimental intoxication consisted of 100 A untwisted filaments rather than the paired helical filaments (PHF) found in the NFT of AD and several other conditions (Down's Syndrome, post-traumatic dementia, etc.). Finally, NFT are not found in dialysis dementia, a condition in which the brain contains a high concentration of Al (Alfrey, LeGendre, & Kaehny, 1976; Burks, Alfrey, Huddlestone, Norenberg, & Lewin, 1976). Here again, it is possible that Al affects only genetically predisposed or otherwise at-risk individuals. Also, the Al content of the CSF of patients with AD has recently been found to be decreased (Delaney, 1979). Perl and Brody (1980) studied hippocampal neurons of AD patients and found that foci of Al were present intracellularly in a high percentage of neurons containing NFT. This finding suggests that simple reliance on cerebral or CSF Al levels may not be a sufficiently sensitive method and that the association between AD and Al deserves further study.

Transmissible agent hypothesis. Cook and Austin (1978) have suggested that familial AD should be thought of as being a transmissible dementia because a spongiform encephalopathy (i.e., a pathology similar to that found in CJD) has been found in a few primates innoculated with brain tissue of familial AD, but not of non-familial AD. It has also been found in a patient whose family members had autopsy-proven AD. Furthermore, it has been ascertained that the pathological changes of AD and spongiform encephalopathy coexist in some patients (Gaches, Supino-Viterbo, & Foncin, 1977). No such evidence exists for non-familial cases except for the finding of DeBoni and Crapper (1978) that paired helical filaments, undistinguishable from those of AD, could be observed in human fetal cerebral neurons 15 to 35 days following injection of brain extract from AD patients.

Sociological and psychological hypotheses. Sociological factors are of course important in AD (as in most other diseases), since the manifestation of dementia is influenced by the social and intellectual status of the patients and of their families. A home sample study conducted in Newcastle-upon-Tyne (Kay, Beamish, & Roth, 1964a)

failed to show any relationship between socioeconomic status and
"organic mental disorders" (including both cerebrovascular disease
and AD). Social isolation was more frequent in the dementia group,
but the authors felt that this was more likely to be a consequence
of the disease rather than its cause. As for the effect of stressful life events, some studies have been negative (Kay, Beamish, &
Roth, 1964a; Oakley, 1965); however, Amster and Krauss (1974) found
that "deteriorated" patients had experienced a greater number of
life crises than controls during the 5 years that preceded the onset
of deterioration. This aspect of the disease certainly deserves
further investigation in view of the known effect of stress on the
immune system (Bartrop, Luchkhurst, Lazarus, Kiloh, & Penny, 1977).
Finally, it has been claimed that patients with senile dementia have
an "obsessive and rigid premorbid personality" (Oakley, 1965). However, the poor definition of patients included in the study makes
the interpretation of this finding difficult. It nevertheless may
be of interest to note that the same claim has been made regarding
Parkinson Disease (Aring, 1962). The complex interactions among
psychosocial factors, depression and dementia have been investigated
in depth by Gurland and his colleagues (Gurland, Dean, Cross, &
Golden, 1980), and have led to the development of a comprehensive
assessment tool (CARE).

The importance of studies such as these cannot be overemphasized.
Even though this is not always appreciated, it is essential when dealing with AD, for either clinical or research purposes, to take into
account not only cognitive changes, but also changes in mental health
and in activities of daily living.

Other Dementias

Multi-infarct dementia (MID) and other (vascular diseases pro-
ducing dementia) (e.g., Binswanger Disease) (Loizou et al., 1981),
are usually related to disease of small intracerebral vessels, which
in turn is often the result of chronic hypertension and/or diabetic
angiopathy. Another vascular mechanism leading to dementia is the
occurrence of repeated attacks of ischemic hypoxia due to inadequate
blood supply. These may cause neuronal loss and gliosis, without
obvious anatomically demonstrable vascular occlusion. Genetic factors also seem to play a significant role in vascular disease (Aakesson, 1969), which tends to affect males more than females. A hereditary form of MID has also been described (Sourander & Walinder,
1977). Other "risk factors" of MID and of dementia in vertebrobasilar insufficiency are reviewed by Rivera and Meyer (1975a). Certainly, multiple infarcts are sometimes found in patients with no
obvious mental deterioration (Fisher, 1968). Clearly, what counts
is not only the absolute amount of infarcted tissue (Roth's "threshold concept"), but the location of the lacunar infarcts; it is said
that dementia is particularly prone to appear when the infarcts af-

fect the thalamic and hypothalamic areas (Castaigne, Buge, Cambier, Escourolle, Brunet, & Degos, 1966).

The etiology of the dementia syndrome of depression in the elderly is quite unclear. Certainly mood change alone does not provide a sufficient explanation because younger depressives, even though they often complain of difficulty in thinking, do not show such a dementia-like picture. Folstein and McHugh (1978) hypothesized that the biochemical abnormalities thought to be present in depression (Schildkraut, 1965) may combine with "the progressive neuronal loss from a variety of causes found in the aging." The genetics of the condition also seem to vary since a positive family history is obtained less often in the dementia syndrome of depression in the elderly than in affective disorders occurring at younger ages.

Diagnostic Considerations

Neurological examination. Aside from the mental status section, the neurological examination of AD patients does not usually show severe abnormalities until the disease is in its most advanced stage. This finding is in keeping with the fact that neuropathological damage tends to be present mainly in the association areas of the cerebral cortex, with a relative sparing of primary motor and sensory cortex. One must recall, however, that the neurological examination of the elderly tends to show considerable changes compared to that of younger adults, and that the majority of these changes are related to disorders of the peripheral organs rather than to acutal CNS changes (Critchley, 1956). The neurological examination of demented patients in a more advanced stage, particularly of those with AD, tends to show more specific abnormalities, especially in terms of gait, posture, and reflexes (Paulson, 1977).

Demented patients, especially those with AD, often exhibit rigidity and/or show abnormal movements such as tremor. Recent work (Boller, Mizutani, Roessman, & Gambetti, 1980) has shown that clinical and neuropathological features of AD are found in up to half of the patients with Parkinson Disease (PD). It has previously been noted that some patients with AD also develop some clinical signs resembling those of PD (Pearce, 1977); however, it is not known how often this occurs, nor whether corresponding subcortical neuropathological changes of PD are found in these AD patients (for a review see Boller, 1982).

The greater occurrence of focal neurological signs is one of the distinguishing features of MID. Similarly, CJD patients show neurological signs in a relatively early stage of the disease. This is usually thought to allow clinical differentiation from AD, but recent work (Watson, 1979) has cautioned that the two conditions may be confused. On the other hand, patients with dementia syndrome

of depression characteristically show no focal abnormality on neurological examination in comparison to age-matched controls.

   Mental status examination and neuropsychological testing. Neuropsychological aspects of dementia have been described extensively.
The major areas of neuropsychological assessment covered by the literature are attention, memory, orientation, language, praxis, visual-
spatial abilities, perception in various modalities, motor and psychomotor skills and higher conceptual and other cognitive abilities.
The following review will be organized according to these categories.

   Attention. Studies of attention in dementia are very few
(Miller, 1981a,b,c). This is unfortunate because making sure that
subjects are attending properly to the tests and to the instructions
is a prerequisite for the interpretation of all neuropsychological
deficits.

   Memory. Patients with dementia do more poorly on memory tasks
than matched controls. The literature indicates that the memory impairment of dementia is global in nature, involving both short-term
and long-term memory in all modalities. Thus, patients with dementia
do not generally have the selective types of amnesia typically seen
in patients with an alcoholic Korsakoff Syndrome (AKS) (Butters &
Cermak, 1980), or patients with limbic system lesions (Milner, 1966,
1968; Scoville & Milner, 1957). Butters and Cermak (1980) suggest
that the memory disorder in dementia may be due to a profound disorder in consolidating and storing new information. This conclusion
is based on the finding that demented patients, unlike AKS patients,
tend not to benefit from various types of cueing or from reduced interference. Furthermore, they do not demonstrate the anterograde-
retrograde gradient typical of AKS, showing instead a global disability in recalling both remote and recent events. Miller (1981a,b;
Miller & Cohen, 1981) concludes that the nature of the memory disorder
in dementia remains unclear, but also points out that both recent and
remote memory appear to be involved. With regard to remote memory,
both Butters and Cermak (1980), and Miller (1981a,b,c) suggest that,
despite the clinical impression that remote memory is preserved in
dementia, objective investigations (Sanders & Warrington, 1971) indicate that remote memory is indeed impaired.

   There are several theoretical explanations concerning the nature
of the memory deficit in dementia. Miller (1981a,b,c) suggests that
disturbed attention or impaired iconic memory reduces the efficiency
with which information is incorporated into short-term memory. Another theory (Warrington & Weiskrantz, 1970) suggests that there is
a disinhibition of the capacity to recall incorrect items. Some investigators have suggested that it is not actually memory that is
impaired, but rather that subjects become more reluctant to report
responses they are unsure about, due to a "criterion shift." This
phenomenon, readily investigated by signal detection analysis, may

be important in elderly depressed individuals. However, there is
some evidence (Miller & Lewis, 1977) that it does not explain the
memory deficit in dementia. Pathological and neurochemical evidence
supporting another attractive theory is presented by Fuld, Katzman,
Davies, and Terry (1982), in relation to a suggestion by Drachman
(1978) that the memory impairment of AD is similar to that produced
in normal young adults by the administration of scopolamine, an anti-
cholinergic. Fuld et al. (1982) showed not only that the presence
of intrusions in mental status and memory test data was related to
the presence of large numbers of senile plaques in the cerebral cortex when tested patients came to autopsy, but also that intrusions
tended to occur in those for whom cholinergic enzymes in the brain
were low. A subsequent double-blind crossover drug study has shown
that intrusions on the Buschke and Fuld (1974) selective reminding
test can be reduced by 43% in AD by the administration of a cholinergic booster (physostigmine and lecithin) in AD patients and that
this reduction is very strongly related to the cholinesterase inhibition measured in cerebrospinal fluid (Thal et al., in press),
documenting the availability of increased acetylcholine to the brain.
Thus, the relationship of intrusions to cholinergic functioning in
AD appears well documented at present.

     In the case of AD, it is often reported that impairment of
memory is among the first signs of the illness (Perez, 1980; Perez,
Rivera, Meyer, Gay, Taylor, & Mathew, 1975). Roth (1980a) has pointed
to the phenomenon of memory impairment for recent events as an early
sign of dementia which often remains the most conspicuous defect during the initial stage of the illness. However, it differs from the
memory deficit found in patients with "pure" amnesic disorders, since
such patients typically have difficulties limited to memory for the
remainder of their lives. Whereas, in the case of the demented patient, the abnormal recent memory deficit gradually merges into more
global intellectual impairment.

     Orientation. Orientation is usually one of the first aspects
of mental status recorded by neurologists and is classically subdivided into orientation for person, place and time. In the initial
and middle stages of dementia, it is unusual for patients to be un-
aware of their own self, but in more advanced stages, patients not
only cannot provide their own name, but also apparently become un-
aware of their own person. This is shown by the fact that they fail
to recognize themselves in a mirror. This failure was apparent in
8 out of 30 demented patients studied by Ajuriaguerra and co-workers
(Ajuriaguerra, Strejilevitch, & Tissot, 1963). Those patients (all
of whom were women with advanced AD except for one who had MID) would
show no evidence of recognition and often would talk to their image
or attempt to touch it as if it were that of another person.

     Disorientation for time is very frequent in subjects with de-
mentia, as well as in those with amnesic syndromes. One might think

that many hospitalized patients tend to lose track of the precise
date, but in a formal study of this problem, Benton, Van Allen, and
Fogel (1964) found that among control patients of Iowa University
Hospital, only very few missed the date by more than one day. By
contrast, among 66 patients with "cerebral damage" (their etiology
is not given in more detail), only 33 (50%) were within one day of
the exact date. In a study that compared AD with HD patients, Kim
and her colleagues (Kim, Morrow, & Boller, 1980) found that AD patients were quite impaired in their orientation for both time and
place. This was in contrast to patients with HD, who were relatively
much better preserved in that particular area of mental status testing. These data suggest that although among demented patients orientation is probably highly correlated with memory and general intellectual functioning, there may occasionally be striking discrepancies
between these various areas of mental status.

   Language. With few exceptions (Wechsler, 1977), demented patients do not show the classical aphasic syndromes found in patients
with focal brain lesions. Nevertheless, language and language-related
difficulties are extremely common in dementia. These consist mainly
of an impoverishment of language, manifested by the use of a limited
vocabulary in narrative speech and impaired verbal fluency. Some
investigators (Albert, Goodglass, Helm, Rubens, & Alexander, 1981),
rather than using the term "aphasia," use such terms as "dementiform
language" or "impaired language performance." Albert et al. (1981)
summarizes the language deficits of dementia as: 1) a breakdown in
logical associations of spoken discourse, resulting in incoherence
of output; 2) a reduction of lexical stock, manifested by naming
deficit; 3) a simplification of syntax; 4) perseverations; 5) echolalia; 6) introduction of improbable or unlikely phrases; 7) tangent-
iality; and, 8) a tendency for the above deficits to increase as
length of conversation increases. A study by Sjogren et al. (1952)
found that anomic disorders are the most common form of language impairment in AD, with fluent aphasia, agraphia and alexia also appearing quite frequently (75%+ of the cases studied). The most prominent
clinical features were reported to be word-finding and comprehension
difficulties, along with perseveration and echolalia. Broca's type
of aphasia is reported to be quite uncommon in AD. This phenomenon
may be related in part to the fact that aging subjects show a much
greater frequency of fluent aphasia than younger ones (Obler, Albert,
Goodglass, & Benson, 1979). In the case of MID, anomic dysphasia is
also quite common, but as would be expected for this illness, language-related symptoms may appear suddenly in the form of a superimposition on the previously existing dementia.

   Rochford (1971) found that the naming difficulty associated with
dementia may be different from what is found in aphasia. Essentially,
the aphasic generally knows what the object to-be-named is, but cannot find the correct word for it, while the demented patient is more
likely to misidentify the object. Demented patients improve their

naming performance when object identification difficulty is minimized, while aphasic patients show no such improvement. The use of a responsive naming task might help in further investigation of this matter.

While Albert et al. (1981) report the presence of comprehension difficulties, it is not clear whether such difficulties are specifically language-related or a product of generalized intellectual impairment. Miller (1981a,b,c) has pointed out that the entire area of language comprehension in dementia has essentially been neglected. This area, plus further investigation of the tendency of demented patients to misidentify objects rather than to develop a specific word-finding disability, appear to merit further study.

Praxis. Apraxia has also been said by Sjogren (1952) to be a frequent finding in AD patients. This is particularly evident when demented patients are asked to perform a series of acts that are to be carried out in sequence in order to achieve a given goal, such as going from cleaning a pipe to filling it, lighting it, and smoking it. This disorder of so-called "ideational apraxia" occurs either because patients do not seem to know how to achieve their goal or because they forget their goal (Heilman, 1979). The behavior of demented patients in classical ideomotor apraxia tasks has not been formally studied.

Visual-spatial abilities and perception. The existence of visual-spatial deficits may be inferred from a number of findings. However, as will be seen, the interpretation of these findings tends to be equivocal. First, there seems to be greater decrement on the performance tests of the Wechsler scales than on the verbal tests (Bolton, Britton, & Savage, 1966; Cleveland & Dysinger, 1944). Since the performance tests tap visual-spatial abilities, one could postulate the presence of a specific decrement in such abilities in persons with dementia. Second, there is more deficit found on progressive matrices tasks than on vocabulatry tasks (Kendrick, Parboosingh, & Post, 1965; Kendrick & Post, 1967; Orme, 1957). Miller (1981a,b,c) reports the results of studies in which demented patients had particular difficulties with mazes and appreciation of reflected space (i.e., dealing with mirror images). Clinically, Joynt and Shoulson (1979) report that demented patients may get lost even in familiar surroundings.

The difficulty with the above considerations is that measures of visual-spatial ability, as well as clinical observation of impaired visual-spatial behavior, are confounded by a number of factors. The relative decrement on performance tests may simply be because performance tests are generally timed, while verbal tests are not. Thus, slowness may be the crucial variable. In addition, spatial disorientation may be associated with sensory impairment, particularly difficulties with vision. In many instances, performance tests are more complex than verbal tests, and difficulty differences in regard to problem solving demands may be the crucial factor (Mack & Carlson, 1978). Miller (1981a,b,c) has suggested that the selective decrement in performance tests may be largely associated with an inability to deal with novel, unfamiliar tasks. Thus, the existence of a specific visual-spatial disorder, such as constructional apraxia or spatial agnosia, is well established; however, the reasons for it may not always be clear and apparent visual-spatial deficits may be secondary to other impairments.

With regard to perception, demented patients appear to have difficulty with the visual identification of objects. A few studies (Ernst, Dalby, & Dalby, 1970a,b; Willanger & Klee, 1966) have reported perceptual distortions during fixation, and abnormalities of a gnostic and praxic nature in a small percentage of demented patients. Also relevant is the finding of Rochford (1971), mentioned above, involving a disturbance of visual recognition in demented patients that diminishes when more familiar and easily recognized stimuli are presented.

The pronounced difficulty of demented patients with performance type visual-spatial tasks has led to the inference that the right hemisphere is more affected by dementia than the left hemisphere, or alternatively put, that the right hemisphere ages more rapidly than the left. Three studies (Birri & Perret, 1980; Goldstein & Shelly, 1981; Gordon & Sim, 1967) have provided some degree of support for this hypothesis, but the data are open to numerous interpretations, and the idea remains controversial. In any event, there is no pathological evidence for greater structural deterioration of the right hemisphere of aged or demented subjects (Roth, 1980a).

Motor and psychomotor skills. The use of motor and psychomotor tests with an elderly population is problematic because of the strong relationship between slowing of motor function and normal aging (Hicks & Birren, 1970). Birren (1964) has stated that "the evidence indicates that all behavior mediated by the central nervous system tends to slow in the aging organism" and "... slowness of behavior is the perceptual manifestation of a primary process of aging in the nervous system." There is no evidence that patients with AD have more impairment of motor or psychomotor function than age matched controls. However, Corkin and colleagues (1981) used a coordinated tapping test and a fine finger movement test as parts of a battery aimed at assessing the effectiveness of lecithin in AD patients. Albert and Kaplan (1980) reported that the sequential motor programming tasks devised by Luria (1966) are useful tests for assessing dementia. Perez, Gay, and Cooke (1978) found a greater right hand-left hand discrepancy in finger tapping speeds in multi-infarct patients than in AD patients. Thus, there appears to be more evidence that AD patients may do relatively well on simple motor tasks as compared to tasks involving bimanual coordination. Miller (1974) found that there is also an impairment of speed of movement execution in the demented, as compared with normal, elderly subjects.

Higher conceptual and cognitive activities. By definition, individuals with dementia have impaired intellectual function and, indeed, in numerous studies demented patients do more poorly on standardized intelligence tests than would be expected, based on the test
norms or in comparison with a normal control group (Miller, 1977;
1981a,b,c). However, for various reasons, while the standard intelligence tests, such as the various Wechsler scales, have demonstrated
the existence of impaired intelligence, they have not been particularly revealing with regard to the specific nature of the intellectual deficit. A major hypothesis has been that dementia is simply
accelerated aging and the same intellectual changes associated with
it are seen chronologically later in nondemented very elderly individuals. This matter has been extensively studied (Goldstein & Shelly,
1975), and the findings are equivocal with some studies supporting
the hypothesis and some not. Factor analysis studies have also been
contradictory, some suggesting a unidimensional intellectual loss,
others finding multidimensional deficit patterns. Whether the intellectual changes found in dementia involve only a single intellectual function or a variety of abilities remains, therefore, an unanswered question. An essentially universal finding is that when one
administers the Wechsler scales or related tests to elderly and/or
demented individuals, both do worse on the performance than on the
verbal tests. According to Miller (1977; 1981a,b,c), there are three
possible explanations for this phenomenon: (1) a speed factor - the
performance tests are timed while the verbal are not; (2) a specific
visual-spatial defect; and, (3) an inability to cope with novel situations. Miller himself accepts the third alternative because the
same phenomenon occurs when speed is not a consideration, and while
demented patients often do have visual-spatial difficulties, there
is an extensive literature documenting marked impairment of acquisition of new information.

In conclusion, even though dementia is associated with impairment of intelligence as measured by IQ tests, IQ tests generally do
not provide sufficiently specific information for elucidation of the
nature of the intellectual deficits seen in various types of dementia.
One solution to this problem has been the application of carefully
selected neuropsychological test batteries consisting of measures of
specific abilities, some having reasonably well understood cerebral
correlates. Table 2 summarizes the neuropsychological tests used by
some investigators in their assessment of dementia.

Differential neuropsychological diagnosis of dementia. Can
neuropsychological tests discriminate among types of dementia, or
between dementia and other forms of neurological disease? While
there have been some studies related to this question, most neuropsychological investigations describe their subjects as having dementia in general, rather than focusing on specific entities such
as AD, MID, etc. Nevertheless, there have been attempts to discriminate among subtypes of dementia using behavioral tests. Some of

Table 2. Batteries used in dementia research.

Gainotti, Caltagirone, Masullo and Miceli (1980)

    1. Word fluency
    2. Phrase construction
    3. Key word memory test
    4. Raven's colored progressive matrices
    5. Immediate visual memory (based on colored matrices material)
    6. Copying designs

Benton, Eslinger and Damasio (1981)

    1. Temporal orientation
    2. Digit span
    3. Digit sequence learning ("Digit supraspan")
    4. Controlled oral word association ("Word fluency")
    5. Logical memory (WMS)
    6. Associate learning (WMS)
    7. Visual retention test
    8. Facial recognition
    9. Judgment of line orientation

Corkin, Growdon, Sullivan, and Shedlack (1981)

    1. Brown-Peterson distractor test
    2. Picture recognition test
    3. Verbal paired-associate learning test (Inglis)
    4. Nonverbal paired-associate learning test
    5. Immediate memory span for digits
    6. Hebb recurring-digits test
    7. Corsi block tapping test
    8. Minnesota test for differential diagnosis of apahsia-counting, naming days, naming pictures, pointing to pictures, pointing to serial items and understanding sentences
    9. Token test
  10. Reporters test
  11. WAIS vocabulary
  12. Gollin incomplete-pictures test
  13. Copying a cube and drawing objects to verbal command
  14. Coordinated tapping test (Thurstone)
  15. Fine finger movement
  16. Apraxia testing (voluntary actions in response to verbal commands)
  17. CARE

Table 2. Batteries used in dementia research (Continued).

Albert and Kaplan (1980)

1. Weschler Adult Intelligence Scale (with additions and special scoring methods).
2. Boston neuropsychological adaptation of the Wechsler Memory Scale.
3. A series of short-term memory tasks utilizing consonant trigrams and words with varying modality (visual vs. auditory) and mode (sequential vs. simultaneous) of presentation.
4. The series of remote memory tests developed by Albert, Butters and Levin (1975); famous faces, recall questionnaire and recognition questionnaire.
5. Parietal-lobe battery: tests of drawing, constructional ability, calculation, right-left orientation and finger localization (Goodglass & Kaplan, 1972).
6. Frontal system battery: tests of motor programming (Luria, 1966), various conceptual abilities, attention, vigilance and verbal fluency. A variety of tests are included in this category including Wisconsin card sorting, Gorham proverbs, Shipley-Hartford scale, Raven's progressive matrices, controlled word association (FAS) and continuous performance tests.

Perez, Gay and Cooke (1978)

1. Wechsler Adult Intelligence Scale
2. Wechsler Memory Scale
3. Finger tapping

these efforts will be reviewed below.

   In a series of papers, Perez and co-workers (Perez, Gay, Taylor, & Rivera, 1975; Perez, Gay, & Taylor, 1975; Perez, Gay, & Cooke, 1978) have shown that it may be possible to discriminate among AD, vertebrobasilar insufficiency and MID with neuropsychological tests. One major finding was that AD patients did significantly worse on the WAIS. A discriminant analysis correctly classified 74% of the subjects into AD and MID categories. Even more powerful findings were obtained with the Wechsler Memory Scale. The discriminant function analysis correctly classified 100% of the cases based on various Wechsler Memory Scale measures. It was also found that the discrepancy between memory and cognitive ability (MQ vs. IQ), was greater in AD than in MID subjects, with memory being more impaired. An additional finding was that the discrepancy in tapping speed between hands was greater in the MID group than in the AD group. In a study

in which a group of patients with vertebrobasilar insufficiency was
also included, it was found thst they did not differ substantially
from the multi-infarct group, although the multi-infarct group did
perform consistently more poorly than the vertebrobasilar insufficiency group. Inspection of the data indicates that while this difference was relatively slight, the difference between the two vascular groups and the AD group was quite striking.

      Gainotti and colleagues (Gainotti, Caltagirone, Masullo, &
Miceli, 1980) compared patients with AD, MID, Normal Pressure Hydrocephalus (NPH), PD, HD, and depression on eight neuropsychological measures. The results of the study were rather complex, involving different patterns of test performance in the different groups.
However, similar to the findings of Perez et al. (1975, 1978), the
AD patients (in this case accompanied by the HD patients) did consistently worse than the other groups. The AD patients were also
particularly impaired on tests of memory and constructional abilities. Butters and Cermak (1980), in an attempt to answer the question of whether there is more than one type of amnesia, discovered
that the pattern of memory disorder found in demented patients was
different from that typically seen in AKS patients. Specifically,
demented patients (in this case individuals with HD), unlike AKS
patients, do not improve their performance under low proactive inhibition conditions or with increased time for rehearsal, nor do
they demonstrate a temporal gradient in recall of remote events.

      Thus far, the differential diagnosis literature offers some
promise that neuropsychological tests can be useful with regard to
discriminating among subtypes of dementia, and in delineating patterns of cognitive dysfunction that may be specifically characteristic of dementia, as opposed to other neurological disorders. However, the work of applying statistically significant group findings
to methods of predicting diagnoses in individual cases remains to
be done.

      There are two major difficulties with research on the neuro-
psychology of dementia: (1) most of the studies have looked at patients at only one point in time. As stated by Miller (1981a,b,c),
"there is a lack of work which systematically tries to follow the
development of cognitive impairments to see how they change with
different stages in the disease process." and (2) patients with
dementia are far from being a homogeneous group. There is a need
to separate patients with AD from those with other types of dementia.
Even then it is probable that among patients with AD, different
patterns of impairment may be found.

Electroencephalography: Spectral Analysis and Evoked Potentials

      The electroencephalogram (EEG) can show changes of a variable

nature in normal elderly. However, they do not occur in all individuals. The most common change in normal aging is slight slowing
of the alpha rhythm. The average occipital frequency around age 70
has decreased from 9.5-10 Hz to 9.0-9.5 Hz, and around 80 years is
8.5-9.0 Hz. Some activity around 8 Hz can also be found. In addition, there is slowing of the waking background rhythm and the appearance of slow waves in the temporal regions, especially on the
left side (Hughes & Cayaffa, 1977; Obrist, 1954, 1976; Obrist &
Henry, 1958; Otomo, 1966).

However, pronounced generalized slowing is uncommon among men-
tally normal subjects with advancing age. In contrast, patients
with dementia generally have rhythms of 7 Hz and below, and the
presence of diffuse theta-delta activity has some correlation with
the clinical picture of dementia (Obrist, 1976; Celesia & Daly,
1977). The EEG is abnormal in virtually all cases of histologically
proven AD (Green, Stevenson, Fonseca, & Wortis, 1952; Gordon & Sim,
1967; Letemendia & Pampiglione, 1958; Liddell, 1958; Nevin, 1970;
Swain, 1959). The primary finding is progressive slowing and disor-
ganizaton of the background pattern. Alpha activity is reduced and
finally disappears, and the tracing shows generalized theta-delta
components. Similar findings can occur in numerous other conditions
(including dementia of other etiologies), and there are no changes
which are specific for AD. Two important points, however, are the
absence of both major focal slowing and paroxysmal activity. The
EEG may be normal in the early stages of the disease.

The EEG, in cerebrovascular disorders, typically shows a somewhat different pattern than that commonly seen in AD. Intermittent
slow wave patterns can occur on one or both sides, and a major focal-
ity can be present. An asymmetrical background pattern with reduction or complete loss of alpha and/or beta activity over one hemisphere may be found. Epileptogenic activity of various forms can
occur, including periodic lateralized epileptiform discharges (PLEDs).
Some alpha rhythm may be retained posteriorly. The above findings
can occur in those cases of cerebrovascular disease leading to intellectual deterioration known as MID (Hachinski, Lassen, & Marshall,
1974).

Although a routine EEG recording cannot differentiate between
organic causes of dementia, a diffusely slow EEG can help to distinguish between organic dementia (if moderate to marked), and a
psychotic reaction to functional origin, such as a depression which
may present as a "pseudodementia." This latter condition is associated with a normal, or only minimally disturbed, EEG pattern.

Numerous EEG and evoked response studies have been performed
in patients with psychosis and an excellent review is available
(Shagass, 1975). Abnormalities in the affective disorders include
faster alpha frequency, prolonged alpha blocking, more fast activity

in power spectrum analysis, evoked response asymmetries, reduced
response amplitudes, etc. However, no findings have been consistent
or specific.

    In early or mild dementia there is considerable overlap and
differentiating patients with mixed symptoms is not an easy task.
Spectral analysis provides a more quantitative assessment of EEG
activity among different frequency ranges, and has been used to
compare the processes of normal aging and dementia (Barlow, 1973;
Marjerrison, Keogy, & Krause, 1969; Muller & Grad, 1970; O'Connor,
Shaw, & Ongley, 1979; Roubicek, 1977). In normal aging there is
a progressive increase of power in the theta band, with a decrease
in power spectrum in patients with dementia vs. patients with depression. The organic group shows higher power in the theta and
delta ranges, while the depressive group shows higher power above
10 Hz. This kind of analysis may offer a means of differentiating
between organic and functional conditions in patients who are diagnostic problems.

    Averaged evoked potentials (AEP) provide an electrophysiologi-
cal correlate of the reception and processing of information. Amplitude and latency of evoked response components provide quantifi-
able measures not obtainable from the routine EEG. Systematic changes
in evoked responses occur with age; for example, latencies of the
early components of the visual response tend to increase after age
65 (Celesia & Daly, 1977). Recent evidence points to differences
among demented patients beyond the normal effects of aging. Interhemispheric differences have been reported among demented patients
(Gersoon, John, Bartlett, & Koenig, 1976). Visual evoked responses
may provide a differentiation of AD from normal aging processes.
Except for the earliest components, AD patients exhibit increased
latency of components as compared with normals (Stam & Op Den Veld,
1978; Visser, Stam, Van Tilburg, Op Den Vester, Blom, & DeRijke,
1976) suggesting a less effective mechanism for the central processing of information. Dementia due to CJD has been associated with
both increased latency and decreased amplitude of components over
time. It is also possible to examine the involvement of brainstem
components in response to auditory stimulation (Chiappa, Gladstone,
& Young, 1979; Stockard, Stockard, & Sharbrough, 1980). Prolongation
of the latency of components occurring during the first ten msec
after stimulation is indicative of organic involvement, although
amplitude differences among individuals seem less reliable as a discriminating factor.

    In conclusion, even though EEG and AEP are not specifically di-
agnostic of various forms of dementia, they are invaluable tools
which provide unique insights into the structural and functional
levels of the brain. In addition, as recently proposed by Kaszniak,
Garron, Fox, Bergen, & Huckman (1979), EEG and AEP may turn out to
be one of the best prognostic indicators of AD and related dementias.

Cerebral Blood Flow (CBF) and Metabolism

Elderly subjects without CNS diseases show normal or only slightly decreased CBF (Dastur, Lane, Hansen, Kety, Butler, Perlin, & Sokoloff, 1963; Lassen & Ingvar, 1980). A reduction of CBF and cerebral metabolism is observed, however, in all the dementias and it correlates with the severity of mental impairment (Fazekas, Alman, & Bessman, 1952; Freyhan, Woodford, & Kefy, 1951; Scheinberg, 1950; Sokoloff, 1961). In early onset AD, there is a marked regional reduction in CBF in the frontal and temporal areas, predominantly in the grey matter (Gustafson & Reisberg, 1974). Patients with MID show a CBF reduction in areas that correspond to the history and clinical localization of the infarcts. They tend to be seen mainly in the territory of either the middle cerebral or vertebrobasilar arteries and only rarely in the territory of the anterior cerebral artery. On occasion, multiple discrete areas of reduced flow are seen (Rivera & Meyer, 1975b). CBF has been found to be decreased in depression as well. Mathew and co-workers (Mathew, Meyer, Francis, Semchuk, Mortel, & Claghorn, 1980), tested 13 patients of mean age 30 with a diagnosis of major depression after a medication washout of 2 weeks. A decrease in CBF was found to be greater in the left hemisphere and correlated well with the severity of depression.

Melamed, Lavy, Siew, Bentin, and Cooper (1978), studied CBF and CT scans of patients with AD and found both decreased CBF, and enlarged ventricles and sulci; however, no correlation between CBF values and the severity of the CT scan changes was found. They concluded that the loss of brain substance is not an important factor in the reduction of CBF in dementia, a conclusion that is in keeping with the finding of decreased CBF in depressed young adults.

A method for adapting the computed tomographic technique to the measurement of local cerebral blood flow is being refined (Gur, Yonas, Wolfson, Kennedy, Drayer, & Gray, 1981). This process is accomplished by recording the x-ray absorption changes due to the presence of the contrast agent gaseous stable Xenon. Rates of diffusion between flowing blood and brain tissue are directly measured during repeat CT scans, while the gas is being inhaled or blown off after a period of inhalation. This information defines blood flow if the blood/tissue partition coefficient is known for the particular region under study. This method can be used to produce maps of regional blood flow in brain slices obtained from the CT technique in which the flow is computed for each voxel (anatomical volume unit) as generated in the CT process. The flow is defined as ml/min/gas of tissue and is displayed by the computer as an anatomical map using a gray or color scale to indicate blood flow in the range <5 - > 110. A unique feature of this method is the calculation of the blood/brain partition coefficient for each voxel at the time of the actual blood flow measurement. This method is particularly well suited to the study of multifocal or diffuse patterns of change, such as may be

seen in degenerative and/or proliferative diseases. Because of the
anatomical resolution, one may expect to detect and be able to localize blood flow changes restricted to nuclear centers or specific
tracts or regions. Moreover, the method is equally precise in deep
and superficial tissues, with respect to both resolution and quantification. Thus, deep thalamic or brainstem changes are as easy to
detect as are those of the cerebral cortex.

In conclusion, even though CBF is not as direct an index of
metabolism as are methods based on glucose utilization (Benson,
Cummings, & Kuhl, 1981), its particular sensitivity to the presence
of cerebral vascular disease may make it the best instrument for the
differential diagnosis of MID from other forms of dementia.

CT Scan Studies

Until less than 10 years ago, in vivo evaluation of cerebral
atrophy and other dementia-related structural brain changes was based
on invasive methods, such as pneumoencephalography and, to a lesser
extent, arteriography. As pointed out by LeMay (1979), some of the
studies performed using these techniques failed to demonstrate a
clear relationship between enlargement of the ventricles and sulci,
and dementia; however, other researchers obtained findings suggesting a correlation between ventricular size and cognitive performance
(Nielsen, Peterson, Thygesen, & Willanger, 1966). Unfortunately,
the complex technology involved in these invasive methods, as well
as unreliable neuropsychological assessments, make it difficult to
evaluate the literature.

The introduction of the CT scan in the early 1970's has made it
considerably easier to perform in vivo evaluations of cerebral structures, and to establish brain and behavior relationships in aging and
demented subjects. To date, three methods have been used for the
purpose of evaluating CT scan data. The most widely used consists
of evaluating the size of the cerebral ventricles and sulci. This
has been carried out in several different ways that include "eye
balling" the CT scan; that is, providing a rough estimate (e.g.,
0 to +++) of atrophy, linear measurements (e.g., measurement of the
width of the frontal horns), perimetric measurements (i.e., area
measurements) and computer based volumetric reconstructions. These
studies (Naeser, Gebhardt, & Levine, 1980; Yamaura, Masatoshi, Kubota,
& Matouzawa, 1980) have found some relationship between CT scan image
and level of cognitive functioning. However, it has also been the
experience of numerous researchers including ourselves (Boller et
al., 1980), that many patients with dementia have no obvious cerebral
atrophy and that some patients with marked cerebral "atrophy" show
no evidence of dementia.

More recently, researchers (Fox, Debrun, Vinuela, Assis, &

Loates, 1979; Naeser et al., 1980; Pullan, Rawcitt, & Isherwood, 1978) have compared patients' cognitive functioning with the "CT Number;" that is, a number related to the coefficient of attenuation of the brain tissue in a given location. One of thes studies (Fox et al., 1979) did not find a clear relationship between brain density on CT scans and dementia. In the other two studies, however, higher CT scan numbers were obtained in nondemented patients than in demented patients. The study by Naeser and colleagues (1980) included a small (N=2) group of patients with depression, and suggested that the CT scan can be of use in the differential diagnosis between depression and dementia, since the two depressed patients had significantly higher CT numbers than the demented patients.

The most recent technique has been introduced by George and his collaborators (George, de Leon, Ferris, & Kreicheff, 1981), and consists of studying gray matter/white matter discriminability. It was found to correlate significantly (P<.05) with estimates of cognitive functioning in patients with AD. In addition, this study found that not all levels of the brain are of equal importance in the assessment of brain changes; the basal ganglia level may be the most descriptive of the changes in AD.

All of the above methods, but especially the latter two, are based on the assumption that dementing illnesses affect not only gray matter, but also white matter; a hypothesis that is certainly compatible with neuropathological data (Terry, 1978a,b). It must be pointed out that even with the newest techniques, there appears to be overlap between the CT scan image of demented and non-demented individuals. This overlap, however, appears to have markedly decreased with the technique of CT scan numbers. Because the techniques mentioned above have been developed quite recently, normative data are not yet available and, therefore, any prospective study including CT scan in the elderly and demented patients must, at the present time, include a series of matched normal controls. Finally, it is possible that serial CT scans will turn out to be of considerable value. There may be more correlation between worsening of dementia over time and evidence of increasing atrophy than has been found so far in "single shot" studies.

Neurochemistry and Neuropharmacology

The finding of altered brain cholinergic transmission in AD has led to many attempts to correct some of its symptoms with drugs aimed at increasing central cholinergic tone. Results so far have been mixed. For example, cholinergic agonists, such as physostigmine, which has been shown to have positive short term effect in AD (Davis, Levy, Rosenberg, Mathe, & Davis, 1982; Davis, Mohs, Davis, Levy, Horvath, Rosenberg, Ross, Rothpearl, & Rosen, 1982; Smith & Swash,

1979), have side effects that make them undesirable for long-term
use. On the other hand, prolonged use of choline and/or lecithin
is safe, although recent studies (Drachman, Glosser, Fleming, &
Longenecker, 1981; Dysken, Fovall, Harris, Noronha, Bergen, Hoeppner,
& Davis, 1981; Etienne, 1981) have found little or no long-term improvements. This could depend on failure to use the optimal dose
of the drugs, too short trial periods, or difficulty with sampling
(Are all subjects really AD? Do all AD patients have the same biochemical disorder?)? Recent attempts (Friedman, Sherman, Ferris,
Reisberg, Bartus, & Schneck, 1981) to combine choline with piracetam
(a cyclic derivative of GABA) have also failed to show significant
cognitive improvements in 10 AD patients. Three of the patients,
however, showed a "marked improvement," and all three had higher
baseline levels of red blood cell (RBC) choline. These results suggest that there may be clinical differences between patients with
different choline levels in RBC and that a biochemical characterization of this type may have important implications as an in vivo diagnostic marker of AD or of certain types of AD.

Neuropathology

Because excellent recent reviews (DeBoni & Crapper, 1978) are
available for AD and MID (Rivera & Meyer, 1975a), neuropathological
findings in dementia will not be reviewed in detail here. One must
emphasize, again, that even autopsies and biopsies (Kaufman &
Catalano, 1979; Moossy, 1969) do not always clearly diagnose and
separate various types of dementia. A sizeable number of demented
patients are found at autopsy to have both AD and vascular changes.
Others show features of both AD and CJD (Ball, 1980; Gaches et al.,
1977), and there are, of course, several instances in which no
specific changes are found (Haase, 1977; Kim, Collins, Parisi,
Wright, & Chu, 1981). Also, there is some suggestion that neuropathology may be different in clinically different types of dementia.
For example, Brun & Gustafson (1978), found that patients with presenile dementia often showed prominent limbic lobe involvement at
autopsy; when during life, a personality disorder had dominated the
picture. They refer to these patients as having Pick's Disease, but
the neuropathological differentiation from AD is not very convincing.

Conclusion: Current Clinical Characterization of Dementias of the Aged

To conclude this review, we will briefly summarize the criteria
usually taken into consideration when diagnosing, in vivo, various
types of "primary" dementia; that is, dementia in which a series of
preliminary tests fail to reveal medical or neurological diseases
that may be responsible.

Alzheimer Disease. At the present time, AD in either its pre-

senile or senile form is usually diagnosed in patients with a characteristic history of progressive memory loss and other cognitive
changes, and an absence of any other disease that could account for
the dementia (Corkin et al., 1981). The progression of the disease
has been subdivided into 3 stages: early forgetfulness stage (mainly
subjective), middle confusional stage (readily apparent to others),
and late dementia stage (in which the patients can no longer take
care of themselves) (Reisberg, Ferris, & Crook, 1981). There are
instances in which the disease is characterized by prominent changes
in affect and personality, and in these cases the pathology may have
a different location (i.e., affecting mainly frontal and limbic
structures) than the typical location (i.e., mainly parietal). In
some cases, "focal" signs (e.g., aphasia, apraxia, etc.), are prominent; but, contrary to what has been stated (Sjogren et al., 1952),
this is not always the case. In the early to middle states, focal
neurological signs, perhaps with the exception of myoclonus (Faden
& Townsend, 1976), are not usually found. Postural and reflex changes
become prominent in later stages of the disease (Paulson, 1977),
which in its terminal stage reduces patients to an often mute vege-
tative state. Conventional EEG and CT scans are often abnormal but
neither these, not other currently available laboratory tests, un-
equivocally establish the diagnosis of AD.

Other Dementias

   Multi-infarct dementia. Hachinski and his collaborators (Hachinski, Lassen, & Marshall, 1974; Hachinski, Iliff, Phil, Zilhka,
Du Boulay, McAllister, Marshall, Russell, & Symon, 1975) have proposed a well known "ischemic score" (which is in turn derived from
Meyer-Gross) (Slater & Roth, 1969) reproduced in Table 3.

   Hypertension, as presumably ascertained by history, as well as
by chest X-Ray and EKG, only receives a score of 1 in Hachinski et
al.'s score, but should probably receive a higher score, since it
is the most important risk factor in MID. A recent study (Rosen,
Terry, Field, Katzman, & Peck, 1980) has shown no overlap between
AD on one hand and MID and "mixed dementia" on the other, using
Hachinski et al.'s score. The number of patients was rather small,
however, and it must be clearly understood that in every day practice,
this score will only differentiate the most "typical" cases of MID
from the "typical" cases of AD; leaving aside the cases where both
pathologies are present (about 20%) (Roth, 1978c). Thus, cases remain where the clinical picture of MID is undistinguishable from AD.
Laboratory tests, such as EEG and CT scan, and especially biochemical tests and the new Xenon enhanced CT scan, may help further reduce
the number of cases where vascular pathology is not predicted in vivo.

   Dementia syndrome of depression. Typically, this syndrome is
diagnosed on the basis of history of functional deterioration, and

Table 3. Ischemic Score

Feature	Score
Abrupt onset	2
Stepwise deterioration	1
Fluctuating course	2
Nocturnal confusion	1
Relative preservation of personality	1
Depression	1
Somatic complaints	1
Emotional incontinence	1
History of hypertension	1
History of strokes	2
Evidence of associated atherosclerosis	1
Focal neurological symptoms	2
Focal neurological signs	2
Total	18

evidence on mental status examination of a "global" disturbance in
the context of clear sensorium (Folstein & McHugh, 1978), usually
with a normal EEG and CT scan. Clearly, all the above criteria are
met by AD as well; therefore, the differential diagnosis often rests
exclusively on follow up and/or response to antidepressant therapy.

In conclusion, as shown in this chapter, many questions remain
concerning the etiology and pathogenesis of AD and related dementias
and there is currently considerable difficulty in reaching a firm
diagnosis, especially in the early stages of the disease. Answers
to these questions can only be provided by a comprehensive longitudinal study that would take into account the various parameters discussed in the preceeding pages.

REFERENCES

Akesson, H.O. A population study of senile and arteriosclerotic
    psychoses. Human Heredity, 1969, 19, 546-566.
Ajuriaguerra, J.D., Strejilevitch, M., & Tissot, R. Apropos de
    quelques conduites devant le miroir de sujets atteints de syn-
    dromes dimentiels du grand age. Neuropsychologia,   1963, 1,
    59-73.
Albert, M.L., Goodglass, H., Helm, M.A., Rubens, A.B., & Alexander,
    M.P. Clinical aspects of dysphasia. New York: Springer-Verlag,
    1981.
Albert, M.L. & Kaplan, E. Organic implications of neuropsychological
    deficits in the elderly. In L.W. Poon, J.L. Fozard, L.S. Cermak,

D. Arenberg, & L. Thompson (Eds.), New directions in memory
and aging. Proceedings of the George A. Talland Memorial Conference. New Jersey: Lawrence Erlbaum Associates, 1980.

Alfrey, A.C., LeGendre, G.R., & Kaehny, W.D. The dialysis encephalopathy syndrome - Possible aluminum intoxication. New England
Journal of Medicine, 1976, 4, 184-188.

Amster, L.E. & Krauss, H.H. The relationship between life crises
and mental deterioration in old age. International Journal of
Aging and Human Development, 1974, 5, 51-55.

Aring, C.D. The riddle of the Parkinson Syndrome. Archives of
Neurology, 1962, 6, 1-4.

Ball, M.J. Features of Creutzfeldt-Jakob Disease in brains of patients with familial dementia of Alzheimer type. Canadian
Journal of Neurological Science, 1980, 7, 51-57.

Barlow, J.S. Autocorrelation and crosscorrelation analysis. In
A. Remond (Ed.), Handbook of electroencephalography and clinical neurophysiology. Amsterdam: Elsevier, 1973.

Bartrop, R.W., Luchkhurst, E., Lazarus, L., Kiloh, L., & Penny, R.
Depressed lymphocyte function after bereavement. Lancet, 1977,
1, 834-836.

Benson, D.F., Cummings, J.L., & Kuhl, D.E. Dementia: Cortical-
subcortical. American Annals of Neurology, 1981, 4, 102.

Benton, A.L., Van Allen, M.W., & Fogel, M.L. Temporal orientation
in cerebral disease. Journal of Nervous and Mental Disease,
1964, 139, 110-119.

Birren, J.E. The psychology of aging. Englewood Cliffs: Prentice
Hall, 1964.

Birri, R. & Perret, E. Differential age effects on left-right and
anterior-posterior brain functions. International Neurological
Society Bulletin, 1980, 3, 13.

Blumenthal, M.D. Chronic organic brain syndromes: Problems and pre-
valence-catchment area 9c-1 (Allegheny County). Draft.

Boller, F., Mizutani, T., Roessmann, U., & Gambetti, P.L. Parkinson
Disease, dementia and Alzheimer Disease: Clinico-pathological
correlations. Annals of Neurology, 1980, 7, 329-335.

Boller, F. Alzheimer's Disease and Parkinson's Disease: Clinical
and pathological association. In B. Reisberg (Ed.), Alzheimer's
Disease and senile dementia. New York: The Free Press, in press.

Bolton, N., Britton, P.G., & Savage, R.D. Some normative data on
the WAIS and its indices in an aged population. Journal of
Clinical Psychology, 1966, 22, 184-188.

Bowen, D.M., Smith, C.B., White, P., & Davidson, A.N. Neurotransmit-
ter-related enzymes and indices of hypoxia in senile dementia
and other abiotrophies. Brain, 1976, 99, 459-496.

Brun, A., & Gustafson, L. Limbic lobe involvement in presenile dementia. Archiv fur Psychiatre und Nervenkrankheiten, 1978,
226, 79-93.

Burks, J.S., Alfrey, A.C., Huddlestone, J., Norenberg, M.D., &
Levin, E. A fatal encephalopathy in chronic hemodialysis
patients. Lancet, 1976, 1, 764-768.

Busse, E. & Blazer, D. The biological and psychological basis of
    geriatric psychiatry. In E. Busse & D. Blazer (Eds.), Handbook
    of geriatric psychiatry. New York: Van Nostrand Reinhold, 1980.
Buschke, H. & Fuld, P.A. Evaluating storage, retention, and retrie-
    val in disordered memory and learning. Neurology, 1974, 24,
    1019-1025.
Butters, N. & Cermak, L.W. Alcoholic Korsakoff's Syndrome: An in-
    formation-processing approach to America. New York: Academic
    Press, 1980.
Castaigne, P., Buge, A., Cambier, J., Escourolle, R., Brunet, P., &
    Degos, J.D. Demence thalamique d'origine vasculaire par ramol-
    lissement bilateral, limite au territoire du pedicule retro-
    mamillaire. Revue Neurologigue, 1966, 114, 89-107.
Celesia, G.G., & Daly, R.F. Effects of aging on visual evoked re-
    sponses. Archives of Neurology, 1977, 34, 403.
Chiappa, K.H., Gladstone, K.J., & Young, R.R. Brainstem auditory
    evoked responses: Studies of waveform variations in 50 normal
    human subjects. Archives of Neurology, 1979, 36, 81.
Cleveland, S. & Dysinger, D. Mental deterioration in senile psy-
    choses. Journal of Abnormal Social Psychology, 1944, 39,
    368-372.
Cook, R.H. & Austin, J.H. Precautions in familial transmissable
    dementia: Including familial Alzheimer's Disease. Archives
    of Neurology, 1978, 35, 697-698.
Corkin, S., Growdon, J.H., Sullivan, E.V., & Shedlack, K. Lecithin
    and cognitive function in aging and dementia. In A. Kidman
    (Ed.), Approaches to nerve and muscle disorders. New York:
    Elsevier, 1981.
Crapper, D.R., Krishman, S.S., & Dalton, A.J. Brain aluminum dis-
    tribution in Alzheimer's Disease and experimental neurofibril-
    lary degeneration. Science, 1973, 180, 511-513.
Crapper, D.R., Krishman, S.S., & Quittkat, S. Aluminum, neurofi-
    brillary degeneration and Alzheimer's Disease. Brain, 1976,
    99, 67-80.
Critchley, M. Neurological changes in the aged. Journal of Chronic
    Diseases, 1956, 3, 459-477.
Dastur, D.K., Lane, M.H., Hansen, D.B., Kety, S., Butler, R., Perlin,
    S., & Sokoloff, L. Effects of aging in cerebral circulation and
    metabolism in man. In J. Birren, R. Butler, S. Greenhouse, L.
    Sokoloff, & M. Yarrow (Eds.), Human aging. Bethesda, MD: PHS
    Publications, 1963.
Davidson, E.A. & Robertson, E.E. Alzheimer's Disease with acne
    roacea in one of identical twins. Journal of Neurology, Neuro-
    surgery and Psychiatry, 1965, 18, 72-77.
Davies, P. & Maloney, A.J. Selective loss of central cholinergic
    neurons in Alzheimer's Disease. Lancet, 1976, 2, 1403.
Davis, B., Levy, M., Rosenberg, G., Mathe, A., & Davis, K. Rela-
    tionship between growth hormone and cortisol and acetycholine:
    A possible neuroendocrine strategy for assessing a cholinergic
    deficit. In S. Corkin, K. Davis, J. Growdon, E. Usdin, & R.

Wurtman (Eds.), Alzheimer's Disease: A report of progress in research. New York: Raven Press, 1982.

Davis, K.L., Mohs, R.C., Davis, B.M., Levy, M.I., Horvath, T.B., Rosenberg, G.S., Ross, A., Rothpearl, A., & Rosen, W. Cholinergic treatment in Alzheimer's Disease: Implications for future research. In S. Corkin, K.L. Davis, J.H. Growdon, E. Usdin, & R.J. Wurtman (Eds.), Alzheimer's Disease: A report of progress in research. New York: Raven Press, 1982.

De Boni, U. & Crapper, D.R. Paired helical filaments of the Alzheimer type in cultured neurons. Nature, 1978, 271, 566-568.

Delaney, J.F. Spinal fluid aluminum levels in patients with Alzheimer disease. Annals of Neurology, 1979, 5, 580-581.

Drachman, D.A. Memory, dementia, and the cholinergic system. In R. Katzman, R.D. Terry, & K.L. Bick (Eds.), Alzheimer's Disease: Senile dementia and related disorders. New York: Raven Press, 1978.

Drachman, D.A., Glosser, G., Fleming, P., & Longenecker, G. Memory decline in the aged: Treatment with high dose lecithin. Neurology, 1981, 31, 101 (abstract).

Dysken, M.W., Fovall, P., Harris, C., Noronha, A., Bergen, D., Hoeppner, T., & Davis, J. Lecithin administration in patients with primary degenerative dementia and in normal volunteers. In S. Corkin, K. Davis, J. Growdon, E. Usdin, & R. Wurtman (Eds.), Alzheimer's Disease: A report of progress in research. New York: Raven Press, 1982.

Ernst, B., Dalby, A., & Dalby, M.A. Aphasic disturbances in presenile dementia. Acta Neurologica Scandinavica Supplement, 1970a, 43, 99-100.

Ernst, B., Dalby, M.A., & Dalby, A. Gnostic praxic disturbances in presenile dementia. Acta Neurologica Scandinavica Supplement, 1970b, 43, 101-102.

Etienne, P., Dastoor, D., Gauthier, S., Ludwick, R., & Collier, B. Lecithin in the treatment of Alzheimer's disease. In S. Corkin, K. Davis, J. Growdon, E. Usdin, & R. Wurtman (Eds.), Alzheimer's Disease: A report of progress in research. New York: Raven Press, 1982.

Faden, A.I. & Townsend, J.J. Myoclonus in Alzheimer Disease - A confusing sign. Archives of Neurology, 1976, 33, 278-280.

Fazekas, J.F., Alman, R.W., & Bessman, A.N. Cerebral physiology of the aged. American Journal of Medical Science, 1952, 223, 245-257.

Fisher, C.M. Dementia in cerebral vascular disease. Cerebral Vascular Diseases: 6th Princeton Conference, 1968, 1, 232-236.

Folstein, M.F. & McHugh, P.R. Dementia syndrome of depression. In R. Katzman, R.D. Terry, & K.L. Bick (Eds.), Alzheimer's Disease: Senile dementia and related disorders. New York: Raven Press, 1978.

Fox, A.J., Debrun, G., Vinuela, F., Assis, L., & Loates, R. Intrathecal metrizamide enhancement of the optic nerve. Journal of Computer Assisted Tomography, 1979, 3, 653-656.

Freyhan, F.A., Woodford, R.B., & Kefy, S.S. Cerebral blood flow and
    metabolism in psychoses of senility. Journal of Nervous and
    Mental Disease, 1951, 113, 449-456.
Friedman, E., Sherman, K.A., Ferris, S.H., Reisberg, B., Bartus, R.,
    & Schneck, M. Clinical response to choline plus piracetam in
    senile dementia: Relation to red-cell choline levels. New
    England Journal of Medicine, 1981, 304, 1490-1491.
Fuld, P.A. Guaranteed stimulus-processing in the evaluation of
    memory and learning. Cortex, 1980, 16, 255-272.
Fuld, P., Katzman, R., Davies, P., & Terry, R. Intrusions as a sign
    of Alzheimer dementia: Clinical and pathological verification.
    Annals of Neurology, 1982, 11, 155-159.
Gaches, J., Supino-Viterbo, V., & Foncin, J.F. Association de mal-
    aches d'Alzheimer et de Creutzfeldt-Jakob. Acta Neurologica
    Belgica, 1977, 77, 202-212.
Gainotti, G., Caltagirone, C., Masullo, C., & Miceli, G. Patterns
    of neuropsychologic impairment in various diagnostic groups of
    dementia. In L. Amaducci, A. Davison, & P. Antuono (Eds.),
    Aging of the brain and dementia. New York: Raven Press, 1980.
Garraway, W.M., Whisnant, J.P., Furlan, A.J., Phillips, L.H., Kurland,
    L.T., & O'Fallon, W.M. The declining incidence of stroke. New
    England Journal of Medicine, 1979, 300, 449-452.
George, A.E., de Leon, M.J., Ferris, S.H., & Kricheff, I.I. Paren-
    chymal CT correlates of senile dementia (Alzheimer Disease):
    Loss of gray-white matter discriminability. American Journal
    of Neurological Research, 1981, 2, 205-213.
Geroon, I.M., John, E.R., Bartlett, F., & Koenig, V. Average evoked
    response (AER) in the electroencephalographic diagnosis of the
    normally aging brain: A practical application. Clinical Elec-
    troencephalography, 1976, 7, 77-91.
Goldstein, G. & Shelly, C. Similarities and differences between
    psychological deficit in aging and brain damage. Journal of
    Gerontology, 1975, 30, 448-455.
Goldstein, G. & Shelly, C. Does the right hemisphere age more rap-
    idly than the left? Journal of Clinical Neuropsychology, 1981,
    3, 65-78.
Gordon, E.B. & Sim, M. Electroencephalogram in presenile dementia.
    Journal of Neurology, Neurosurgery and Psychiatry, 1967, 30,
    285.
Gottfries, C.G., Gottfries, I., & Roos, B.E. The investigation of
    homovanillic acid in the human brain and its correlation to
    senile dementia. British Journal of Psychiatry, 1969a, 115,
    563-574.
Gottfries, C.G., Gottfries, I., & Roos, B.E. Homovanillic acid and
    5-hydroxyin-doleacetic acid in the cerebrospinal fluid of
    patients with senile dementia, presenile dementia and Park-
    insonism. Journal of Neurochemistry, 1969b, 16, 1341-1345.
Green, M.A., Stevenson, L.D., Fonseca, J.E., & Wortis, S.B. Cere-
    bral biopsy in patients with presenile dementia. Diseases of
    the Nervous System, 1952, 13, 303-307.

Gur, D., Yonas, H., Herbert, D., Wolfson, H.D., Kennedy, S., Drayer, B.P., & Gray, J. Xenon enhanced dynamic computed tomography: Multilevel cerebral blood flow studies. Journal of Computer Assisted Tomography, 1981, 5, 334-340.

Gurland, B., Dean, L., Cross, P., & Golden, R. The epidemiology of depression and dementia in the elderly: The use of multiple indicators of these conditions. In J.O. Cole & J.E. Barrett (Eds.), Psychopathology in the aged. New York: Raven Press, 1980.

Gustafson, L. & Reisberg, J. Regional cerebral blood flow related to psychiatric symptoms in dementia with onset in the presenile period. Acta Psychiatrica Scandinavica, 1974, 50, 516-538.

Haase, G.R. Diseases presenting as dementia. In E. Wells (Ed.), Dementia. Philadelphia: Davis, 1977.

Hachinski, V.C., Lassen, N.A., & Marshall, J. Multi-infarct dementia: A cause of mental deterioration in the elderly. Lancet, 1974, 2, 207-209.

Hachinski, V.C., Iliff, L.D., Phil, M., Zilhka, E., Du Boulay, G.H., McAllister, V., Marshall, J., Russell, R., & Symon, L. Cerebral blood flow in dementia. Archives of Neurology, 1975, 32 632-637.

Heilman, K.M. Apraxia. In K.M. Heilman & E. Valenstein (Eds.), Clinical neuropsychology. New York: Oxford University Press, 1979.

Heston, L.L. Alzheimer's Disease, trisomy 21, and myeloproliferative disorders: Associations suggesting a genetic diathesis. Science, 1977, 196, 322-323.

Heston, L.L. Alzheimer's Disease and senile dementia: Genetic relationships to Down's syndrome and hematologic cancer. Research Publications of the Association for Research in Nervous and Mental Disease, 1979, 57, 167-176.

Heston, L.L. & Mastri, A. The genetics of Alzheimer's Disease - Associations with hemotalogic malignancy and Down's Syndrome. Archives of General Psychiatry, 1977, 34, 976-981.

Heston, L.L. & White, J. Pedigrees of 30 families with Alzheimer Disease: Associations with defective organization of microfilaments and microtubules. Behavior Genetics, 1978, 8, 315-331.

Heyman, A. Differentiation of Alzheimer's Disease from multi-infarct dementia. In R. Katzman, R.D. Terry, & K.L. Bick (Eds.), Alzheimer's Disease: Senile dementia and related disorders. New York: Raven Press, 1978.

Hicks, L.H. & Birren, J.E. Aging, brain damage and psychomotor slowing. Psychological Bulletin, 1970, 74, 377-396.

Hughes, J.R. & Cayaffa, J.J. The EEG in patients at different ages without organic cerebral disease. Electroencephalography and Clinical Neurophysiology, 1977, 42, 776-784.

Hunter, R., Dayan, A.D., & Wilson, J. Alzheimer's Disease in one monozygotic twin. Journal of Neurology, Neurosurgery and Psychiatry, 1972, 35, 707-710.

Ishii, T. & Haga, S. Immunoelectron microscopic localization of

immunoglobulins in amyloid filuli of senile plaques. Acta
Neuropathologica, 1976, 36, 243-260.

Joynt, R.V., & Shoulson, I. Dementia. In K.M. Heilman & E. Valenstein (Eds.), Clinical neuropsychology. New York: Oxford University Press, 1979.

Kaszniak, A.W., Garron, D., Fox, J.H., Bergen, D., & Huckman, M.
Cerebral atrophy, EEG slowing, age, education and cognitive
functioning in suspected dementia. Neurology, 1979, 29, 1273-
1979.

Katzman, R., Terry, R.D., & Bick, K.L. Recommendations of the nos-
ology, epidemiology, and etiology and pathophysiology commis-
sions of the workshop-conference on Alzheimer's disease - senile
dementia and related disorders. In R. Katzman, R.D. Terry, &
K.L. Bick (Eds.), Alzheimer's Disease: Senile dementia and related disorders. New York: Raven Press, 1978.

Katzman, R., & Karasu, T.B. Differential diagnosis of dementia.
In W.S. Fields (Ed.), Neurological and sensory disorders in
the elderly. New York: Stratton, 1975.

Katzman, R. The prevalence and malignancy of Alzheimer Disease.
Archives of Neurology, 1976, 33, 217-218.

Kaufman, H.H. & Catalano, L.W. Diagnostic brain biopsy: A series
of 50 cases and a review. Neurosurgery, 1979, 4, 129-136.

Kay, D.W., Beamish, P., & Roth, M. Old age mental disorders in
Newcastle-upon-Tyne Part II: A study of possible social and
medical causes. British Journal of Psychiatry, 1964, 110,
146-158.

Kendrick, D.C., Parboosingh, R.C., & Post, F. A synonym learning
test for use with elderly psychiatric subjects: A validation
study. British Journal of Social and Clinical Psychology,
1965, 4, 63-71.

Kendrick, D.C. & Post, F. Differences in cognitive status between
healthy, psychiatrically ill, and diffusely brain-damaged
elderly subjects. British Journal of Psychiatry, 1967, 113,
75-81.

Kim, Y., Morrow, L., & Boller, F. Patterns of intellectual impairment in Alzheimer's and Huntington's diseases. International
Neurological Society Bulletin, 1980, 3, 20-21.

Kim, R.C., Collins, G.H., Parisi, J.E., Wright, A.W., & Chu, Y.B.
Familial dementia of adult onset with pathological findings
of a "non-specific" nature. Brain, 1981, 104, 61-78.

Larsson, T., Sjogren, T., & Jacobson, G. Senile dementia: A clinical sociomedical and genetic study. Acta Psychiatrica
Scandanavica Supplement 167, 1963, 39, 1-259.

Lassen, N.A. & Ingvar, D.H. Blood flow in the aging normal brain
and in senile dementia. In L. Amadvcci, A. Davison, & P.
Antuono (Eds.), Aging of the brain and dementia. New York:
Raven, Press, 1980.

LeMay, M. The radiologic investigation of dementia and cerebral
atrophy. In S. Wolpert (Ed.), Central nervous system: Approaches to radiologic diagnosis. New York: Grune & Stratton,

1979.

Letemendia, F. & Pampiglione, G. Clinical and electroencephalographic observations in Alzheimer's Disease. Journal of Neurology, Neurosurgery and Psychiatry, 1958, 21, 167-172.

Liddell, D.W. Investigations of EEG findings in presenile dementia. Journal of Neurology, Neurosurgery and Psychiatry, 1958, 21, 173-176.

Loizou, L.A., Kendall, B.E., & Marshall, J. Subcortical arteriosclerotic encephalopathy: A clinical and radiological investigation. Journal of Neurology, Neurosurgery and Psychiatry, 1981, 44, 294-304.

Luria, A.R. Higher cortical functions in man. New York: Basic Books, 1966.

Mack, J.L. & Carlson, J. Conceptual deficits and aging: The category test. Perceptual and Motor Skills, 1978, 46, 123-128.

Marjerrison, G., Keogy, R.P., & Krause, A.E. Quantitative analysis of the EEG in psychopathological states: Human experimental and clinical observations. Electroencephalography and Clinical Neurophysiology, 1969, 27, 676.

Marsden, C.D. & Harrison, M.J. Outcome of investigation of patients with presenile dementia. British Medical Journal, 1972, 2, 249-252.

Mathew, R.J., Meyer, J.S., Francis, D.J., Semchuk, K.M., Mortel, K., & Claghorn, J.L. Cerebral blood flow in depression. American Journal of Psychiatry, 1980, 137, 1449-1450.

Matthews, W.B. & Will, R.G. Epidemiology of Creutzfeldt-Jakob Disease in Britain. Neurology, 1982, 32, A186.

McDermott, J.R., Smith, A.I., Iqbal, K., & Wisniewski, M. Aluminum and Alzheimer's Disease. Lancet, 1977, 2, 710-711.

Melamed, E., Lavy, S., Siew, F., Bentin, S., & Cooper, G. Correlation between regional cerebral blood flow and brain atrophy in dementia. Journal of Neurology, Neurosurgery and Psychiatry, 1978, 41, 894-899.

Miller, E. Abnormal aging. London: Wiley, 1977.

Miller, E. The differential psychological evaluation. In N.E. Miller & G.D. Cohen, (Eds.), Clinical aspects of Alzheimer's Disease and senile dementia. New York, Raven Press, 1981a.

Miller, E. The nature of the cognitive deficit in senile dementia. In N.E. Miller & G.D. Cohen (Eds.), Clinical aspects of Alzheimer's Disease and senile dementia. New York: Raven Press, 1981b.

Miller, E. The nature of the cognitive deficit in senile dementia. In N.E. Miller & G.D. Cohen (Eds.), Clinical aspects of Alzheimer's Disease and senile dementia. New York: Raven Press, 1981c.

Miller, N.E. & Cohen, G.D. Clinical aspects of Alzheimer's Disease and senile dementia: Synopsis and future perspectives in assessment, treatment, and service delivery. In N.E. Miller & G.D. Cohen (Eds.), Clinical aspects of Alzheimer's Disease and senile dementia. New York: Raven Press, 1981.

Miller, E. & Lewis, P. Recognition memory in elderly patients with depression and dementia: A signal detection analysis. Journal of Abnormal Psychology, 1977, 86, 84-86.

Milner, B. Amnesia following operation on the temporal lobes. In C. Whitty & O. Zangwill (Eds.), Amnesia. London: Butterworths, 1966.

Milner, B. Visual recognition and recall after right temporal-lobe excision in man. Neuropsychologia, 1968, 6, 191-209.

Moossy, J. Diagnostic cerebral biopsy. In J.F. Toole (Ed.), Special techniques for neurologic diagnosis. Philadelphia: F.A. Davis Co., 1969.

Mortimer, J.A. Epidemiological aspects of Alzheimer's Disease. In F.J. Pirozzolo & G.S. Mali (Eds.), The aging nervous system. New York: Praeger, 1980.

Mortimer, J.A. & Schuman, L.M. The epidemiology of dementia. New York: Oxford University Press, 1981.

Muller, H.F. & Grad, B. EEG, biochemical and behavioral characteristics of elderly psychiatric patients. Electroencephalography and Clinical Neurophysiology, 1970, 27, 409-413.

Naeser, M.A., Gebhardt, C., & Levine, H.L. Decreased computerized tomography numbers in patients with presenile dementia. Archives of Neurology, 1980, 37, 401-409.

Nandy, K. Brain-reactive antibodies in aging and senile dementia. In R. Katzman, R.D. Terry, & K.L. Bick (Eds.), Alzheimer's Disease: Senile dementia and related disorders. New York: Raven Press, 1978.

Neuman, M.A. & Cohn, R. Progressive subcortical gliosis, a rare form of presenile dementia. Brain, 1967, 90, 405-418.

Nevin, S. Alzheimer's Disease. CIBA Foundation Symposium, 1970, 89-93.

Nielsen, R., Peterson, O., Thygesen, P., & Willanger, R. Encephalographic cortical atrophy, relationship to ventricular atrophy and intellectual impairment. Acta Radiologica, 1966, 4, 437-448.

Nishimura, T., Harigrichi, S., & Tada, K. Changes in brain water-soluble proteins with presenile and senile dementia. Excerpta Medica, 1975, 2, 139-142.

O'Connor, K.P., Shaw, J.C., & Ongley, C.O. The EEG and differential diagnosis in psychogeriatrics. British Journal of Psychiatry, 1979, 135, 156-162.

Oakley, D.P. Senile dementia - Some etiological factors. British Journal of Psychiatry, 1965, 111, 414-419.

Obler, L.K., Albert, M., Goodglass, H., & Benson, D. Aphasia type and aging. Brain and Language, 1978, 6, 318-322.

Obrist, W.D. The electroencephalogram of normal aged adults. Electroencephalography and Clinical Neurophysiology, 1954, 6, 235-244.

Obrist, W.D. Problems of aging. In A. Remond (Ed.), Handbook of electroencephalography and clinical neurophysiology. Amsterdam: Elsevier, 1976.

Obrist, W.D. & Henry, C.E. Electroencephalographic findings in aged psychiatric patients. *Journal of Nervous and Mental Disease*, 1958, 126, 254-267.

Orme, J.E. Non-verbal and verbal performance in normal age, senile dementia and elderly depression. *Journal of Gerontology*, 1957, 12, 408-413.

Otomo, E. Electroencephalography in old age: Dominant alpha pattern. *Electroencephalography and Clinical Neurophysiology*, 1966, 21, 489-491.

Paulson, G.W. The neurological examination in dementia. In C.E. Wells (Ed.), *Dementia*. Philadelphia: Davis, 1977.

Pearce, J. Symptomatic Parkinsonism. *Postgraduate Medicine Journal*, 1977, 53, 726-728.

Perez, F.I. Behavioral studies of dementia: Methods of investigation and analysis. In J.O. Cole & J.E. Barrett (Eds.), *Psychopathology in the aged*. New York: Raven Press, 1980.

Perez, F.I., Gay, J.R., & Cooke, N.A. Neuropsychological aspects of Alzheimer's Disease and multi-infarct dementia. In K. Nandy (Ed.), *Senile dementia: A biomedical approach*. Amsterdam: Elsevier, 1978.

Perez, F.I., Gay, F.R., & Taylor, R.L. WAIS Performance of neurologically impaired aged. *Psychological Reports*, 1975, 37, 1043-1047.

Perez, F.I., Gay, J.R., Taylor, R.L., & Rivera, V.M. Patterns of memory performance in the neurologically impaired aged. *Canadian Journal of Neurological Sciences*, 1975, 2, 347-355.

Perez, F.I., Rivera, V.M., Meyer, J.S., Gay, J.R., Taylor, R.L., & Mathew , N.T. Analysis of intellectual and cognitive performance in patients with multi-infarct dementia, vertebrobasilar insufficiency with dementia and Alzheimer's disease. *Journal of Neurology, Neurosurgery and Psychiatry*, 1975, 38, 533-540.

Perl, D.P., & Brody, A.R. Alzheimer's Disease: X-ray spectrometric evidence of alumin accumulation in neurofibrillary tangle-bearing neurons. *Science*, 1980, 208, 297-299.

Perry, E.K., Gibson, P.H., Blessed, G., Perry, R.H., & Tomlinson, B.E. Neurotransmitter enzyme abnormalities in senile dementia. *Journal of Neurological Science*, 1977, 34, 247-265.

Perry, E.K., Perry, R.H., Blessed, G., & Tomlinson, B.E. Necropsy evidence of central cholinergic deficits in senile dementia. *Lancet*, 1977, 3, 1891

Perry, E.K., Tomlinson, B.E., Blessed, G., Bergmann, K., Gibson, P.H., & Perry, R.H. Correlation of cholinergic abnormalities with senile plaques and mental test scores in senile dementia. *British Medical Journal*, 1978, 2, 1457-1459.

Pullan, B.R., Rawcitt, R.E., & Isherwood, I. Tissue characterization by analysis of the distribution of attenuation values in computed tomography scans: A preliminary report. *Journal of Computer Assisted Tomography*, 1978, 2, 49-54.

Reisberg, B., Ferris, S., & Crook, T. Signs, symptoms and course of age-associated cognitive decline. In S. Corkin, K. Davis, J. Growdon, E. Usdin, & R. Wurtman (Eds.), *Alzheimer's Disease: A* report of progress in research. New York: Raven Press, 1982.

Reisine, T.D., Yamamura, H.I., Bird, E.D., Spokes, E., & Enna, S.J. Pre and postsynaptic neurochemical alterations in Alzheimer's disease. Brain Research, 1978, 159, 477-481.

Rivera, V.M. & Meyer, J.S. Dementia and cerebrovascular disease. In J.S. Meyer (Ed.), Modern concepts of cerebrovascular disease. New York: Spectrum, 1975.

Rochford, G. A study of naming errors in dysphasic and in demented patients. Neuropsychologia, 1971, 9, 437-443.

Rosen, W.G., Terry, R.D., Fuld, P.A., Katzman, R., & Peck, A. Pathological verification of ischemic score in differentiation of dementias. Annals of Neurology, 1980, 7, 486-488.

Roth, M. The psychiatric disorders of later life. Psychiatric Annals, 1976, 6, 417-445.

Roth, M. Diagnosis of senile and related forms of dementia. In R. Katzman, R.D. Terry, & K.L. Bick (Eds.), Alzheimer's Disease: Senile dementia and related disorders. New York: Raven Press, 1978.

Roth, M. Epidemiological studies. In R. Katzman, R.D. Terry, & K.L. Bick (Eds.), Alzheimer's Disease: Senile dementia and related disorders. New York: Raven Press, 1978b.

Roth, M. Discussion. In R. Katzman, R.D. Terry, & K.L. Bick (Eds.), Alzheimer's Disease: Senile dementias and related disorders. New York: Raven Press, 1978c.

Roth, M. Aging of the brain and dementia: An overview. In L. Amaducci, A. Davison, & P. Antuono (Eds.), Aging of the brain and dementia. New York: Raven Press, 1980a.

Roth, M. Senile dementia and its borderlands. In J.O. Cole & J.E. Barrett (Eds.), Psychopathology in the aged. New York: Raven Press, 1980b.

Roubicek, J. The electroencephalogram in the middle-aged and the elderly. Journal of the American Geriatric Society, 1977, 25, 145-152.

Sanders, H.I. & Warrington, E.K. Memory for remote events in amnesic patients. Brain, 1971, 94, 661-668.

Scheinberg, P. Cerebral blood flow in vascular disease of the brain. American Journal of Medicine, 1950, 8, 139-147.

Schildkraut, J.J. The catecholamine hypothesis of affective disorders. A review of supporting evidence. American Journal of Psychiatry, 1965, 122, 509-522.

Scoville, W.B. & Milner, B. Loss of recent memory after bilateral hippocampal lesions. Journal of Neurology, Neurosurgery and Psychiatry, 1957, 20, 11-21.

Shagass, C. EEG and evoked potentials in the psychoses. In D. Freedman (Ed.), Biology of the major psychoses. New York: Raven, Press, 1975.

Sjogren, T., Sjogren, H., & Lindgren, A.G. Morbus Alzheimer and morbus Pick: A genetic, clinical and patho-anatomical study. Acta Psychiatrica et Neurologica Scandanavica Supplement, 1952, 82, 1-152.

Slater, E. & Roth, M. Ageing and the mental diseases of the aged.
    In Mayer Gross Clinical Psychiatry. London: Bailliere Tindall
    and Cassell, 1969.

Smith, C.M. & Swash, M. Physotigmine in Alzheimer's disease.
    Lancet, 1979, 1, 42.

Sokoloff, L. Cerebral circulation and metabolism changes associated
    with aging. Research Publications of the Association for Re-
    Nervous and Mental Disease, 1961, 41, 237-254.

Sourander, P. & Walinder, J. Hereditary multi-infarct dementia:
    Morphological and clinical studies of a new disease. Acta
    Neuropathologica, 1977, 39, 247-254.

Stam, F.C. & Op Den Velde, W. Haptoglobin types in Alzheimer's
    Disease and senile dementia. In R. Katzman, R.D. Terry, &
    K.L. Bick (Eds.), Alzheimer's Disease: Senile dementia and
    related disorders. New York: Raven Press, 1978.

Stockard, J.J., Stockard, J.E., & Sharbrough, F.W. Brainstem audi-
    tory evoked potentials in neurology: Methodology, interpreta-
    tion, clinical application. In M. Aminoff (Ed.), Electrodiag-
    nosis in clinical neurology. New York: Churchill Livingstone,
    1980.

Swain, J.M. Elctroencephalographic abnormalities in presenile
    atrophy. Neurology, 1959, 9, 722-727.

Terry, R.D. Ultrastructural alterations in senile dementia. In R.
    Katzman, R.D. Terry, & K.L. Bick (Eds.), Alzheimer's Disease:
    Senile dementia and related disorders. New York: Raven Press,
    1978a.

Terry, R.D. Senile dementia. Federal Proceedings, 1978b, 37,
    2837-2840.

Thal, L., Fuld, P., Masur, D., & Sharpless, N. Oral physostigmine
    and lecitchin improve memory in AD. Annals of Neurology, in
    press.

Visser, S.L., Stam, F.C., Van Tilburg, W., Op Den Velde, W., Blom,
    J.L., & DeRijke, W. Visual evoked response in senile and pre-
    senile dementia. Electroencephalography and Clinical Neuro-
    physiology, 1976, 40, 385-392.

Walford, R.L. General immunology of aging. In B.L. Strehler (Ed.),
    Advances in gerontological research. New York: Academic Press,
    1967.

Ward, B.E., Cook, R.H., Robinson, A., & Austin, J.H. Increased
    aneuploidy in Alzheimer disease. American Journal of Medical
    Genetics, 1979, 3, 137-144.

Warrington, E.K. & Weiskrantz, L. Amnesic syndrome: Consolidation
    or retrieval? Nature, 1970, 228, 628-630.

Watson, C.P. Clinical similarity of Alzheimer and Creutzfeldt-
    Jakob disease. Annals of Neurology, 1979, 6, 368-369.

Wechsler, A.F. Presenile dementia presenting as aphasia. Journal
    of Neurology, Neurosurgery and Psychiatry, 1977, 40, 303-305.

Wells, C.E. Chronic brain disease: An overview. American Journal
    of Psychiatry, 1978, 135, 1-12.

White, P., Hiley, C.R., & Goodhardt, M.J. Neocortical cholinergic neurons in elderly people. <u>Lancet</u>, 1977, <u>2</u>, 668-681.

White, B.J., Crandall, C., Goudsmit, J., Morrow, C.H., Alling, D.W., Gajdusek, D.C., & Tijio, J.H. Cytogenetic studies of familial and sporadic Alzheimer disease. <u>American Journal of Medical Genetics</u>, 1981, <u>10</u>, 77-89.

Willanger, R. & Klee, A. Metamorphopsia and other visual disturbances with latency occurring in patients with diffuse cerebral lesions. <u>Acta Neurologica Scandinavica Supplement</u>, 1966, <u>42</u>, 1-18.

Yamaura, H., Masatoshi, I., Kubota, K., & Matouzawa, T. Brain atrophy during aging: A quantitative study with computed tomography. <u>Journal of Gerontology</u>, 1980, <u>35</u>, 492-498.

MEMORY ASSESSMENT: EVIDENCE OF THE HETEROGENEITY OF AMNESIC SYMPTOMS[1]

Nelson Butters[1], Patti Miliotis[1], Marilyn S. Albert[2], and Daniel S. Sax[3]

Boston Veterans Administration Medical Center and Boston University School of Medicine[1], Massachusetts General Hospital[2], Boston University School of Medicine[3], Boston, Massachusetts

It is well known to even fledgling clinical neuropsychologists that memory disorders are ubiquitous after brain damage and that standardized tests exist for documenting the presence and severity of these memory deficits. Severe impairments in the learning of new information and in the recall of public and personal events from the remote past occur after head trauma, long-term alcohol abuse, strokes, encephalitis, bilateral ECT, and as an early sign of progressive dementing illnesses. Tests such as the Wechsler Memory Scale and the Benton Visual Retention Test have proven valuable, but not perfect, tools for the assessment of these problems.

Despite this awareness of memory impairments, most neuropsychologists have been insensitive to the multidimensional nature of the symptoms. Usually implicitly, but sometimes explicitly, it has been assumed that all debilitating memory deficits, regardless of etiology, may be treated as a single symptom or cognitive problem. Amnesic patients with bilateral hippocampal lesions and patients with medial diencephalic damage have often been treated as two exemplars of a single underlying clinical entity. In recent years this situation has changed as evidence has accumulated that the "amnesias" are as heterogeneous as the "aphasias" and the "apraxias". Based upon studies from several laboratories, it now appears that there are important qualitative differences among the anterograde and retrograde memory deficits of various neurological populations. While failures in retention and recall following diencephalic and hippocampal lesions may have some superficial similarities, close scrutiny has shown these amnesic populations to have distinctive patterns of deficits when a broad range of memory capacities are assessed. Similarly,

direct comparisons of the memory deficits of amnesic and demented
patients have uncovered differences which may be of some importance
in making prognostic and rehabilitative judgments.

The main purpose of this chapter will be to emphasize the heterogeneity of the anterograde and retrograde memory disorders of amnesic and demented patients. We wish not only to convince the reader
of the clinical importance of a thorough memory assessment, but also
to illuminate the ongoing symbiotic relationship between experimental
and clinical neuropsychology. The discovery that memory tests are
among the most sensitive psychometric instruments for distinguishing
among various patient populations has evolved from "basic" research
into brain-behavior relationships. Although it may be fashionable
for some neuropsychologists to label themselves as "experimental" or
"clinical," it is hoped that the data reviewed here will demonstrate
that such divisions are both artificial and unrewarding.

Comparisons of Anterograde/Retrograde Memory Deficits of Amnesics

Since amnesia has been associated with numerous etiologies (e.g.,
alcohol, vascular, viral, traumatic) and brain sites (e.g., diencephalon, hippocampus), it is important to determine whether all amnesias
reflect identical underlying impairments or whether with sensitive
neuropsychological evaluations amnesic populations can be shown to
differ in their anterograde and retrograde memory deficits. Warrington and her collaborators (Baddeley & Warrington, 1970; Warrington &
Weiskrantz, 1973; Warrington, 1981) have championed the position that
amnesia is a unitary disorder, regardless of the etiology or anatomical basis of the disease. Their investigations of amnesia have included patients with alcoholic, viral, anoxic and surgical etiologies,
and they report that all their patients have performed similarly on
their various learning and cognitive tasks. All of their amnesic patients obtained normal scores on short-term memory tasks, were highly
sensitive to proactive interference and exhibited the same encoding
strategies.

Lhermitte and Signoret (1972) compared patients with alcoholic
Korsakoff's syndrome and postencephalitic (herpes simplex) patients
on a battery of four memory tasks and reached a conclusion at variance with that of Warrington and her collaborators. On a task requiring the learning and memory of a spatial array, the alcoholic
Korsakoff patients showed better retention than did the postencephalitic patients; whereas on tests involving the learning of a verbal
sequence, a logical arrangement and a code, the postencephalitic patients were superior to the alcoholic Korsakoff patients. Since the
neuropathology of Korsakoff's syndrome (Victor, Adams, & Collins,
1971), and herpes encephalitis (Drachman & Adams, 1962; Drachman &
Arbit, 1966) involve the midline diencephalon and the mesial portions
of the temporal lobes respectively, Lhermitte and Signoret's (1972)

findings may be viewed as the first systematic attempt to differentiate "diencephalic" and "hippocampal" amnesia (Squire, 1981). This
topic will occupy the focus of our attention at a later point in this
chapter.

Important distinctions between the memory disorders of alcoholic
Korsakoff and postencephalitic patients were also noted in a previous
report (Butters, 1979). While the alcoholic Korsakoff patients were
severely impaired on short-term memory (STM) tests using the Brown-
Peterson (Peterson & Peterson, 1959) distractor technique, all four
of the postencephalitic patients tested scored within the normal range
on this task. When both groups were administered the retrograde amnesia battery developed by Albert, Butters and Levin (1979), the retrograde anmesia of the postencephalitic patients appeared to be more
severe than that of the alcoholic Korsakoff patients, and revealed
less of a temporal gradient in which very remote memories are relatively spared.

This double dissociation between alcoholic Korsakoff and postencephalitic patients on tests of short-term memory and retrograde
amnesia not only emphasizes possible differences among amnesic populations, but also suggests that anterograde and retrograde amnesic
symptoms may not necessarily be correlated (Benson & Geschwind, 1967).
The capacities to acquire new information and to recall past events
may depend upon different neuroanatomical structures and psychological processes. Fedio and Van Buren's (1974) demonstration that anterograde and retrograde verbal memory deficits may be separated by
stimulation along the anterior-posterior axis of the left temporal
lobe is consistent with the above noted behavioral dissociations.

During the past two years, Squire and Cohen (Squire & Cohen,
1981; Cohen & Squire, 1981; Squire, 1981), Goldberg and his associates (Goldberg, Antin, Bilder, Gerstman, Hughes, & Mattis, 1981),
as well as some published (Albert, Butters, & Brandt, 1981a,b) and
unpublished data from our laboratory, have provided further evidence
for both the independence and the variability of anterograde and retrograde memory losses. Cohen and Squire (1981) administered seven
different tests of remote memory to alcoholic Korsakoff patients, depressed patients receiving bilateral ECT and to the extensively studied amnesic patient, N.A. (Teuber, Milner, & Vaughan, 1968; Squire
& Slater, 1978; Squire & Moore, 1979), who became amnesic for verbal
materials in 1960 following a stab wound to the brain with a fencing
foil. A recent CT scan study (Squire & Moore, 1979) has shown N.A.'s
lesion to be located in the vicinity of the dorsomedial thalamic nucleus of the left hemisphere. Although N.A. and the two patient
groups were severely impaired on verbal paired-associate and recall
testing, they differed significantly in their performance on the tests
of remote memory. Patient N.A. and the ECT patients had relatively
brief retrograde amnesias (2-4 years), while the Korsakoff patients'
loss of remote memory extended over several decades, and was charac-

terized by a temporal gradient in which very remote memories (e.g., from the 1930's and 1940's) were relatively spared.

Based upon the report that Brenda Milner's famous patient (H.M.) with bilateral hippocampal lesions also has a very limited loss of memories prior to his operation (Scoville & Milner, 1957; Milner, 1966, 1970), Cohen and Squire (1981) concluded that the retrograde amnesias of alcoholic Korsakoff patients and those of other amnesic patients are quite distinct and involve different memory and cognitive impairments. They suggested that brief retrograde memory losses are typical when amnesia results from lesions restricted to the diencephalon or hippocampus, and that the extended retrograde losses of alcoholic Korsakoff (and postencephalitic) patients represent the superimposition of additional brain damage and subsequent cognitive difficulties on an amnesic syndrome. The neuroradiological evidence (Lishman,1981; Carlen, Wilkinson, Wortzman, Holgate, Cordingley, Lee, Huzar, Moddel, Singh, Kiraly, & Rankin, 1981) that long-term alcohol abuse is associated with marked atrophy of cortical, as well as diencephalic, structures is consistent with this conclusion. Furthermore, the demonstration that long-term non-Korsakoff alcoholics may have remote memory losses that are qualitatively similar to those of alcoholic Korsakoff patients (Albert, Butters, & Brandt, 1980), suggests that the retrograde amnesia of the Korsakoff patients may be partially an artifact of a progressive anterograde amnesia. If alcoholics learn less and less each year during their 20 to 30 year hsitories of alcohol abuse, it is not surprising that the retrograde amnesia of alcoholic Korsakoff patients extends over many decades and is characterized by a steep temporal gradient.

Goldberg et al. (1981) have also demonstrated, in a case report of a traumatic amnesia, the separation of anterograde and retrograde amnesic symptoms. Their 36 year old male patient had an open skull fracture in the right temporoparietal region resulting in extensive damage to the mesial and lateral surfaces of the right temporal lobe and to the ventral tegmental area of the upper mesencephalon. Although the patient had severe anterograde and retrograde amnesia immediately following his injury in 1977, his anterograde, but not retrograde amnesia, evidenced marked improvement during the next two years. In the 18 month period separating his two evaluations, the patient's MQ improved from 86 to 106, and a corresponding increment was seen on a complex verbal recall test (Buschke's Selective Reminding Task), whereas his severely impaired performance on Albert et al's. (1979) retrograde amnesia battery remained almost unchanged. Thus, two years following his trauma and subsequent surgery, the patient was able to learn new information, but was unable to recall public or personal events that occurred prior to his accident. Since damage to the right temporal lobe had not been associated previously with a general loss of old memories, Goldberg et al. (1981) suggested that the tegmental lesion was responsible for their patient's inability to recall remote public events. They hypothesized that selective

mesencephalic reticular activation of limbic structures is essential
for retrieval of information from long-term storage.

Our comparative studies of the retrograde amnesias of selected
amnesic patients also supports the thesis that anterograde and retrograde amnesias are separable and that patient populations may be differentiated by the qualitative and quantitative characteristics of
their impairments in remote memory. Figures one and two show the
performance of 10 alcoholic Korsakoff patients, 20 normal control
subjects and of amnesic patients S.S. and R.B. on two paired-associate learning tasks. The alcoholic Korsakoff patients are similar
to those described in previous reports from this laboratory (Butters
& Cermak, 1980). Their 20-30 year histories of alcohol abuse and
malnutrition had resulted in chronic amnesic syndromes sufficient to
require their institutionalization. At the time of testing, the
Korsakoff patients had a mean age of 55 years, a mean verbal IQ (WAIS)
of 106, and a mean MQ (WMS) of 76.

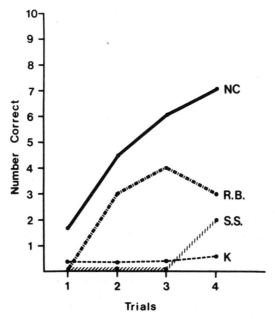

Fig. 1.   Performance of alcoholic Korsakoffs (K), normal controls
          (NC) and patients S.S. and R.B. on a verbal-verbal paired-
          associate task.

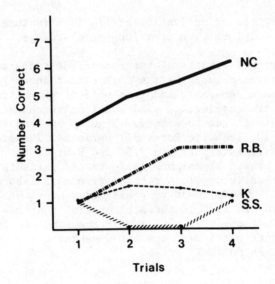

Fig. 2. Performance of alcoholic Korsakoffs (K), normal controls (NC) and patients S.S. and R.B. on a symbol-digit paired-associate task.

Patient S.S. has been described previously in great detail (Cermak, 1976). He is a 54 year old optical engineer whose amnesia dates from 1971 when he contracted herpes encephalitis. Despite an IQ (WAIS) of 130 and an MQ (WMS) of 90, S.S. cannot remember every-day events for more than a few minutes and is unable to recall public or personal events that occurred prior to his infection. R.B. is a 49 year old male computer designer who developed amnesic symptoms in 1981 following the clipping of an anterior communicating artery an-eurysm. In the weeks following surgery he was observed to have in-ordinate difficulty in retaining new information, although his mem-ory for events prior to this surgery seemed to be relatively intact. At the time of testing, his IQ (WAIS-R) was 141 and his MQ (WMS) was 97. Due to their anterograde memory disorders, neither patient was able to resume his occupation and had to be maintained in a highly supervised environment. The similar patterns of IQ-MQ scatter for S.S., R.B. and the alcoholic Korsakoff patients should be stressed because much of the data to be presented will demonstrate that, des-pite this psychometric equivalence, the patients differed signifi-cantly in the nature of their memory deficits.

The normal controls have a mean age of 54 years. Although IQ
scores are not available for this group, it should be noted that
their educational attainment (mean: 11.4 years of formal education)
was similar to that of the alcoholic Korsakoff patients (mean: 12.2
years), but was far below the levels completed by S.S. (18 years of
education) and R.B. (18 years of education). Since educational level
and performance on memory tasks are usually highly correlated, the
differences between patients S.S. and R.B. and the control group are
likely understated.

It is evident in Figures 1 and 2 that the alcoholic Korsakoff
patients, and patients S.S. and R.B., are severely impaired in their
attempts to learn new information. Figure 1 shows the results for
a verbal paired-associate task in which the subjects had to learn 10
difficult word associations (e.g., neck-salt). The results for a
symbol-digit paired-associate learning task are presented in Figure
2. On this latter test, the subjects had to associate seven geo-
metric symbols with single-digit numbers, so that whenever a symbol
was exposed, the subjects would provide the appropriate number.
While the normal control subjects evidenced steady improvement (i.e.,
learning) over the four trials of each task, the alcoholic Korsakoff
patients, S.S. and R.B., demonstrated limited improvement between
trials 1 and 4.

The performance of the amnesic patients and control subjects
were compared on a verbal short-term memory task using the Brown-
Peterson (Peterson & Peterson, 1959) distractor techniques. On each
trial the subjects were read four words and then asked to count back-
ward from a three-digit number (e.g., 100) by three's until the examiner said "stop." After 15 or 30 seconds of such counting (i.e.,
distraction), the examiner stopped the subjects and asked them to recall the four words that had just been presented. The results for
the alcoholic Korsakoff patients and patient S.S. are consistent with
previous reports (Butters & Cermak, 1975; Cermak, 1976; Butters,
1979), using less demanding STM tests; that is, word triads or consonant trigrams as the to-be-recalled materials. Despite their similar performances on the paired-associate tasks, presented in Figure
3, the alcoholic Korsakoff patients and patient S.S. performed differently on the four-word STM test. While the alcoholic Korsakoff
patients were able to recall few words after either delay interval,
the postencephalitic patient S.S. remembered as many words as the
normal controls, even after 30 seconds of distractor activity. R.B.,
who actually performed somewhat better than S.S. on the two paired-
associate tasks, manifested a precipitous decline in recall between
the 15 and 30 second delay intervals.

This lack of correspondence between performance on paired-associate and STM tasks is deserving of further comment. Squire and
Slater (1978), using the Brown-Peterson (Peterson & Peterson, 1959)
distractor procedure, reported that patient N.A. was severely impaired

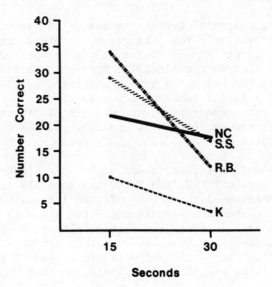

Fig. 3.   Performance of alcoholic Korsakoffs (K), normal controls
          (NC) and patients S.S. and R.B. on a Brown-Peterson short-
          term memory task with 15- and 30-second delays.

in his ability to retain verbal information beyond a few seconds.
Given the highly localized nature of N.A.'s lesion in the region of
the dorsomedial thalamic nucleus of the left hemisphere (Squire &
Moore, 1979), it would appear that damage to midline diencephalon
was sufficient to produce significant impairments in STM. However,
deficits on the Brown-Peterson distractor tasks have also been reported in brain-damaged patients without amnesic syndromes. Patients
with lesions involving the right parietal lobe have shown rapid loss
of visually presented verbal and nonverbal materials (Samuels, Butters
& Goodglass, 1971), especially if the stimuli were initially exposed
to the patients' left visual field. Another study reported that both
left and right temporal lobectomies (with relatively little involvement of the hippocampus) were followed by auditory verbal deficits
on the Brown-Peterson tasks (Samuels, Butters & Fedio, 1972).
Warrington and her colleagues (Warrington & Shallice, 1969, 1972;
Shallice & Warrington, 1970; Warrington, Logue & Pratt, 1972) described auditory verbal STM deficits in three nonamnesic patients
with damage to the posterior parietal cortex of the left hemisphere.
These patients had a reduced auditory (but not visual) immediate
memory span for letters and numbers which could not be reduced to a
motor speech impairment of a problem with auditory perception. When
a patients' STM was assessed with the Brown-Peterson technique,

strings of one, two or three letters were forgotten more rapidly
after auditory than following visual presentation. Despite this
severe impairment in immediate and STM, these patients' long-term
memory appeared intact, as evidenced by their normal performance on
verbal paired-associate and recall tasks. In view of this evidence
(i.e., that cortical lesions can be associated with modality-specific
STM deficits), the attribution of all of an anmesic patients' problems on distractor tasks to diencephalic or hippocampal lesions remains problematical. It is possible that some of the STM deficits
of alcoholic Korsakoff patients, and of patients N.A. and R.B., may
be due to cortical damage which accompanies the diencephalic-limbic
lesions responsible for the patients' deficits on paired-associate
learning tasks.

    To determine whether the alcoholic Korsakoff patients R.B. and
S.S. differed significantly in their capacity to recall remote events,
their performances on an up-dated version of Albert et al.'s (1979)
Famous Faces Test and Public Events Recall Questionnaire were com-

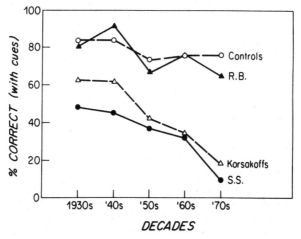

Fig. 4. Performance of alcoholic Korsakoffs, normal controls and
         patients S.S. and R.B. on Albert et al.'s (1979) Famous
         Faces Test.

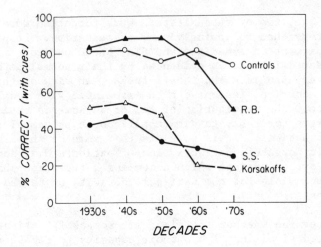

Fig. 5. Performance of alcoholic Korsakoffs, normal controls and
         patients S.S. and R.B. on Albert et al.'s (1979) Recall
         Questionnaire of Public Events.

pared. The Famous Faces Test consists of 188 photographs of famous
individuals from the 1920's to 1980. The photographs are divided
into six decades with approximately 30 pictures in each group. An
individual was assigned to the decade in which he or she first became well-known to the public at large. If subjects have difficulty
in identifying a given face, a set of phonemic and semantic cues are
given alternately. The Public Events Recall Questionnaire consists
of 148 questions regarding public events and people famous between
1920 and 1980. There are 24 or 25 questions for each decade, and
again phonemic and sematic cues are available if a subject has difficulty with uncued recall.

     The results of the Famous Faces Test and the Public Events Re-
call Questionnaire are shown in Figures 4 and 5. It is evident that
despite the similarity of the patients' performance on paired-associate learning (i.e., anterograde amnesia), they demonstrated remarkable differences in their ability to recall events preceding the onset of their illness. Since S.S. had been amnesic since 1971, his
performance on faces and questions from the 1970's should be considered as evidence of his anterograde, not his retrograde, amnesia.
Both the alcoholic Korsakoff patients and patient S.S. manifested
severe retrograde amnesias which extended over many decades. While

a relative sparing of public events and famous faces from the 1930's
and 1940's is evident for S.S., as well as the Korsakoff patients,
S.S.'s performance on both tests was somewhat more impaired and
"flatter" than that of the alcoholic Korsakoff patients. This difference became more striking when it was considered that S.S.'s IQ
was 30 points higher than that of the Korsakoff patients and that he
had six more years of formal education.

It is the performance of R.B. that most clearly demonstrated
the independence of anterograde and retrograde amnesia. This electrical engineer who was severely impaired on the two paired-associate
learning tasks had little difficulty on either the Famous Faces Test
or the Public Events Recall Questionnaire. On the faces test, he did
not differ from the normal controls. On the recall test, he encountered some difficulty with events from the 1970's, but had no problems
remembering events and people from 1930 to 1970. Of all our patients,
R.B. best exemplified the so-called brief RA described by Cohen and
Squire (1981), as typical of amnesic patients like H.M. (Scoville &
Milner, 1957; Milner, 1966,1970), and N.A. (Squire & Slater, 1978;
Squire & Cohen, 1981; Cohen & Squire, 1981).

If one accepts the premise that retrograde amnesia, in its pure
form, is usually very brief, how shall we explain the extended and
severe losses of the alcoholic Korsakoff patients and of postencephalitic patients like S.S.? As noted previously, it has been suggested (Butters & Albert, 1981; Squire & Cohen, 1981) that some of the
alcoholic Korsakoff patients' loss of remote memories may be arti-
factual. Since long-term alcoholics may retain somewhat less information each year due to a chronic learning deficit (Ryan & Butters,
1980), their store of remote memories for the recent past may be
mildly or moderately deficient. If some acute forgetting (or other
cognitive problem) appears during the Wernicke stage of the illness,
and is superimposed on the alcoholic patients' already deficient
store, a severe retrograde amnesia with a temporal gradient might be
expected. There is evidence that this model may have some validity
for the alcoholic Korsakoff patient (Albert, Butters & Brandt, 1980),
but it obviously cannot account for the severe memory loss of patients
like S.S. Since postencephalitics do not approach the acute onset of
their disorder with a deficient store of information, their retrograde amnesia must reflect a general retrieval difficulty or a pervasive degrading and loss of old memories. The fact that the retrograde amnesia of S.S. and other psotencephalitics tends to be "flat"
(i.e., equivalent for all decades) does not allow us to choose between these two alternatives.

Another unresolved issue is the remarkable contrast between the
retrograde amnesias of postencephalitic patients like S.S., and of
patient H.M. Because the memory problems of both H.M. and postencephalitic patients have been attributed to bilateral destruction
of the hippocampi within the mesial temporal region (Scoville &

Milner, 1957; Milner, 1966,1970; Drachman & Adams, 1962; Drachman & Arbit, 1966), one might anticipate that their memory disorders would be quantitatively and qualitatively similar. However, unlike the limited loss of remote memories reported for H.M., all of the post-encephalitic patients evaluated with Albert et al.'s (1979) Famous Faces Test and Public Events Recall Questionnaire have been found to have severe retrograde amnesias involving several decades of their lives (Butters, 1979; Butters & Cermak, 1980). One possible explanation for this difference may involve the extent of hippocampal and temporal lobe damage. If anterograde and retrograde amnesias are separable along the anterior-posterior axis of the temporal lobes (Fedio & Van Buren, 1974), then it is possible that S.S. and other postencephalitic patients have more extensive (and posterior) temporal lobe damage than does H.M. The fact that postencephalitic patients often have mild aphasic disorders certainly suggests that their lesions extend more posteriorly and laterally than H.M.'s anterior and mesial surgical ablation. Presumably, the more posterior the lesion, the more severe the patient's retrograde amnesia may be.

While the studies reviewed to this point have been concerned primarily with the separation of anterograde and retrograde amnesias, investigations of the forgetting of newly acquired information have shown that the anterograde amnesias associated with hippocampal and diencephalic lesions or dysfunction may involve different underlying processes. Huppert and Piercy (1977, 1978, 1979) have reported that when H.M., alcoholic Korsakoff patients, and normal control subjects attain the same level of learning, important differences emerge in their rates of forgetting over a seven day period. These investigators showed each subject 120 slides of colored pictures photographed from magazines. The subjects' recognition memory for these pictures was tested 19 minutes, one day, and seven days later. During each recognition test, 40 of the original (i.e., previously exposed) slides and 40 new (i.e., not previously exposed) slides were presented in a random order, and the subjects were asked to indicate with a yes or no response whether they had seen each slide before. To insure that all subjects would attain approximately the same level of learning at the 10-minute delay period, exposure time during the initial presentation of the slides was manipulated to insure a performance level of at least 75% correct. For the normal control group, each slide had to be exposed for only one second to attain this 75% level after a 10 minute delay; for the amnesic patients, exposure times of four to eight seconds were necessary to attain this level of correct recognition. Thus, by providing additional time for inspection, it was possible to produce significant improvement in the learning of the amnesic patients.

The results of Huppert and Piercy's (1977, 1978, 1979) studies showed that recognition performance declined with increasing retention intervals (one day, seven days) for the normal control subjects, H.M., and the alcoholic Korsakoff patients. Although the rate of

decline did not differ for the normal control group and the alcoholic
Korsakoff patients over this seven day period, H.M.'s performance revealed a much steeper rate of forgetting time than did the scores of
the other two groups. Huppert and Piercy suggested, on the basis of
their results, that the anterograde amnesias of H.M. and the alcoholic
Korsakoff patients involved different deficits in information processing. The alcoholic Korsakoff patients' difficulties may have emanated from a lack of stimulus analysis or encoding. When provided
with sufficient time to fully analyze a complex stimulus, these patients were capable of learning, and demonstrated normal recognition
over an extended period of time. H.M.'s rapid decline in recognition
cannot, however, be accounted for by such a cognitive deficit. Huppert and Piercy (1977, 1978, 1979) postulated that H.M.'s difficulty
in learning new materials may also have reflected a deficit in stimulus analysis, but that his inability to retain newly learned material may have been an indicator of an additional problem with consolidation and storage.

        Squire (1981) evaluated patient N.A., alcoholic Korsakoff pa-
tients, and depressed patients receiving ECT on pictorial and verbal
forgetting tasks similar to the ones used by Huppert and Piercy.
Following the presentation of 120 photographs of colored pictures
(or sentences), yes-no recognition tests were administered after 10-
minute, two-hour, and 32-hour delays. Each recognition test consisted of 80 pictures (or sentences). Forty of the 80 stimuli were
drawn from the original 120 exposed pictures (or sentences) while
the other 40 were distractor items that had not been presented before.
For each of the 80 pictures (or sentences), the subjects were asked
to indicate whether the stimulus had been exposed previously. To insure that the patient groups would perform as well as the normal control subjects on the 10-minute recognition test, the 120 pictures (or
sentences) were exposed to patients for four or eight seconds and to
normal control subjects for only one second.

        The results of Squire's (1981) forgetting study are consistent
with Huppert and Piercy's (1977, 1978, 1979) findings and conclusions.
Patient N.A., whose lesion was reported to be limited to the midline
thalamus (Squire & Moore, 1979), and alcoholic Korsakoff patients,
whose critical lesion was also supposed to involve the medial diencephalon (Victor et al., 1971), did not differ from normal controls
in their rate of forgetting. In contrast, the patients receiving
ECT evidenced a rapid decay of verbal and pictorial material during
the 32-hour period, despite the fact that all groups performed equiv-
alently on the 10-minute recognition task. Based upon his data and
those of Huppert and Piercy, Squire proposed that ECT affects memory
by disrupting hippocampal mechanisms concerned with the consolidation
process. He also concluded that amnesic symptoms associated with diencephalic and hippocampal dysfunction were dissociable in terms of
the stage of information processing adversely affected.

    The results of this forgetting task are shown in Figure 6.
While the alcoholic Korsakoff patients' forgetting curve was essentially identical to that of the normal controls, the performances of
S.S. and R.B. indicated that these amnesic patients forgot pictorial
information at a rate faster than normal. After a 10 minute delay,
S.S.'s recognition was slightly poorer than that of the normals, but
on the six-hour recognition test S.S. and the normal control subjects
performed similarly. On the seven-day recognition test, however,
S.S.'s inability to retain previously acquired pictorial information
was clearly revealed. Normal control subjects recognized an average
of 27.14 pictures, whereas S.S.'s recognition score of 22 was only
slightly above chance performance. R.B.'s recognition performance
after 10-minute and six-hour delays was actually superior to the performance of the control subjects, but after seven days he and the
control subjects did not differ in their recognition performance.
The steepness of R.B.'s forgetting curve between the six-hour and
seven-day testing sessions served as a testimonial to his inability
to retain newly acquired information in a normal fashion.

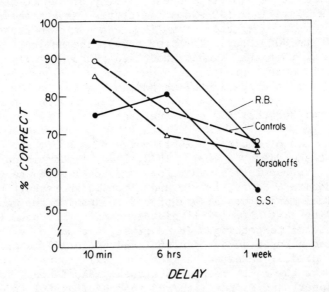

Fig. 6. Forgetting of pictures: Percentage of pictures correctly
         recognized after 10-minute, 6-hour, and 7-day delays by
         alcoholic Korsakoffs, normal controls, and patients S.S.
         and R.B.

In view of the demonstrated involvement of diencephalic structures in alcoholic Korsakoff's disease (Victor et al., 1971), and
of the hippocampus in herpes encephalitis (Drachman & Adams, 1962),
our findings for S.S. and the alcoholic Korsakoff patients must be
viewed as consistent with Huppert and Piercy's (1977, 1978, 1979)
and Squire's (1981) data, and supportive of their thesis that amnesias following hippocampal and diencephalic damage are behaviorally
dissociable. Our data may also provide some clues as to the neuroanatomical structures involved in R.B.'s amnesic condition. Although
amnesic symptoms following the clipping of anterior communicating
artery aneurysms have been noted previously (Lindqvist & Norlen,
1966), the neuroanatomical substrates of this disorder remain a mys-
tery. However, the fact that both H.M. and R.B. displayed severe
learning impairments, limited retrograde amnesias and rapid forgetting of pictorial materials was sufficient reason to question whether
the clipping of the anterior communicating artery can directly or indirectly (e.g., via damage to the septal nuclei) affect the integrity
of the hippocampi.

In summary, the present findings provide two forms of evidence
that amnesia is not a unitary disorder. One, amnesic patients with
similar psychmetric profiles on standardized intelligence and memory
tests have been shown to differ in their pattern of learning, retrieval and forgetting deficits depending upon the etiology of their disease and the locus of their brain damage. Two, careful testing has
revealed differences between the anterograde and retrograde memory
deficits of these patients. It appears now that the ability to learn
new information and to recall remote events may depend upon different
anatomical structures and cognitive processes. The implications of
these findings for the diagnostic functions of clinical neuropsychologists are obvious. A complete description of a patient's memory
symptoms and prognosis requires more than is provided by our current
arsenal of standardized memory tests. We shall undoubtedly witness
the emergence of comprehensive memory batteries to fill this need,
and it is most likely that these "new" clinical tests will draw
heavily upon some of the experimental techniques we have described.
From our perspective, the evidence of the heterogeneity of amnesic
symptoms also underlines the indivisibility of clinical and experimental neuropsychology.

COMPARISONS OF THE MEMORY DISORDERS OF PATIENTS WITH ALCOHOLIC KOR-
SAKOFF'S SYNDROME AND PATIENTS WITH HUNTINGTON'S DISEASE

Severe memory disorders are not unique to amnesic patients. In
fact, complaints regarding memory (anterograde and retrograde) are
among the first symptoms of progressive dementing disorders (Miller,
1977). The major difference between pure amnesia and progressive
dementia is that the memory loss of the demented patient is part of

a broader intellectual decline. Although the amnesic patient's IQ
usually remains within the normal range, despite his severely impaired memory quotient, both the IQ and the MQ of the demented patient decline progressively as the illness advances. IQ and MQ
scores in the 80's are common relatively early in the dementing process. Given the previously cited evidence of the diversity of amnesic symptoms, it is of some interest as to whether the severe memory disorders of amnesic and demented patients involve the same underlying processes.

Several studies (Butters, Tarlow, Cermak, & Sax, 1976; Butters
& Grady, 1977; Meudell, Butters, & Montgomery, 1978; Oscar-Berman &
Zola-Morgan, 1980a,b; Albert, Butters, & Brandt, 1981a,b), comparing
the memory disorders of alcoholic Korsakoff patients and patients
with Huntington's Disease (HD), have indicated that these patients'
anterograde and retrograde memory deficits are distinguishable.
Patients with Huntington's Disease have a genetically transmitted
disorder which results in a progressive atrophy of the basal ganglia
and cerebral cortex. Their most common behavioral symptoms include
involuntary choreic movements and a progressive dementia in which
severe memory problems form an integral part of the broader intellectual decline (Caine, Ebert, & Weingartner, 1977). Since these
previous investigations have been reviewed in detail elsewhere
(Butters, Albert, & Sax, 1979; Butters & Cermak, 1980), we shall
discuss them briefly and then concentrate more fully upon some recent findings concerned with the nonverbal and pictorial memory
capacities of HD and Korsakoff patients.

On Brown-Peterson (Peterson & Peterson, 1959) distractor tasks,
HD patients perform as poorly as do patients with alcoholic Korsakoff's disease, but the role of interference, encoding and rehearsal
in this deficit is less apparent for the HD patients (Butters et al.,
1976; Butters & Grady, 1977; Meudell et al., 1978). Manipulations
of proactive interference (PI) and rehearsal time can improve the
Korsakoff patients' performance on distractor tasks, but such changes
in experimental conditions have virtually no effect upon the HD
patients' ability to recall materials presented 18 or 20 seconds previously. Although the results of these investigations do not reveal
the specific nature of the HD patients' anterograde memory deficits,
they do suggest that these patients have difficulty storing new information (i.e., a deficit in consolidation). The HD patients' failure to improve with low PI conditions, and with increased time for
rehearsal, is consistent with the notion that these patients may lack
some of the neuroanatomical structures necessary for consolidating
and then storing new information.

Oscar-Berman and Zola-Morgan (1980a,b) have compared alcoholic
Korsakoff and HD patients on a series of visual and spatial discrimination tasks. In the initial experiment (Oscar-Berman & Zola-Morgan,
1980a), visual and spatial reversal learning tests were administered.

While the Korsakoff patients were impaired on both types of reversal problems, the HD patients had difficulty only with the visual reversals. An inspection of the types of errors compiled on the visual tasks suggested that the HD and Korsakoff patients' deficiencies involved different learning, cognitive and motivational mechanisms. In a second experiment (Oscar-Berman & Zola-Morgan, 1980b), the Korsakoff and HD patients learned a series of two-choice simultaneous and concurrent pattern discriminations. Again, both patient groups were impaired, but they differed in the nature of their deficits. The HD patients were equally impaired on simultaneous and concurrent discriminations, whereas the Korsakoff patients encountered more difficulty with the concurrent than with the simultaneous tests. In summarizing their findings, Oscar-Berman and Zola-Morgan (1980b) suggested that although both groups of patients were deficient in their ability to form stimulus-reinforcement associations, the Korsakoff, but not the HD, patients' deficiencies also involved an increased sensitivity to proactive interference and a lack of sensitivity to reinforcement contingencies.

To determine whether the HD patients also differed from the alcoholic Korsakoff patients in their ability to recall people and public events from the remote past, Albert et al.'s (1979) remote memory battery was administered to the alcoholic Korsakoff and the HD patients (Albert et al., 1981a). Like the alcoholic Korsakoff patients, the HD patients were severely impaired in their ability to identify famous people and recall public events, but their retrograde amnesia was not characterized by a temporal gradient in which famous faces and public events from the 1930's and 1940's were relatively spared. That is, the HD patients had as much difficulty with faces and events from the 1930's and 1940's as faces and events from the 1960's and 1970's. Wilson, Kaszniak and Fox's (1981) report of very similar results for patients with senile dementia of the Alzheimer's type suggests that "flat" retrograde amnesias may be associated with a number of dementing illnesses.

In a second study, Albert et al. (1981b) compared the performances of advanced HD (diagnosed three to seven years prior to testing), and recently diagnosed HD (less than 12 months prior to testing) patients on their remote memory battery. The recenlty diagnosed HD patients, who showed only a mild cognitive loss at this early stage of the disease, had a retrograde amnesia which was quantitatively less severe, but qualitatively similar, to that of the advanced patients. Like the advanced HD patients, the recently diagnosed HD patients' impairments in the identification of remote events and famous faces extended equally over all decades of their lives. On the basis of these results for the recently diagnosed HD patients, Albert et al. (1981b) concluded that the "flat" retrograde amnesia, which seems to characterize all stages of the disease, cannot be attributed to the dementing process per se. They also noted that the equal loss of remote memories over all time periods sampled was con-

sistent with the thesis that these patients had a storage deficit
affecting both the consolidation of new memory traces and the maintenance of engrams formed prior to the onset of the disease.

Our most recent studies have focused on the nonverbal and pictorial memory capacities of HD patients. The impetus for these investigations emanated from the findings of Dricker, Butters, Berman,
Samuels and Carey (1978), who employed a series of facial recognition
and matching tasks to evaluate the role of stimulus analysis in the
learning deficits of alcoholic Korsakoff patients and of patients
with right hemisphere damage. Their results indicated that since
the Korsakoff and right hemisphere patients were impaired on a simultaneous, facial matching-to-sample task, the patients' failures
to recognize faces could not be attributed totally to a memory problem. Further analyses suggested that the patients' difficulty in
matching faces was due to their tendency to analyze and equate faces
on the basis of superficial piecemeal cues (e.g., hair color or styl-
ing), instead of the configurational relationships among the eyes,
nose and mouth. Dricker et al. (1978) proposed that such inadequate
stimulus analysis served as the foundation for the patients' inability to remember faces and other patterned stimuli.

Given Dricker et al.'s (1978) findings, our recent studies with
HD patients have explored three issues. One, do HD patients have an
impairment for face recognition equivalent to those noted for amnesic
Korsakoff and right hemisphere patients? Two, if severe memory deficits are found in HD patients, can they be attributed to incomplete
or partial stimulus analysis? Three, if the HD patients, like the alcoholic Korsakoff and right hemisphere patients, fail to analyze all
of the relevant features of faces, can orientation tasks designed to
encourage a complete analysis of facial features ameliorate the matching and recognition skills of any of these patient groups? To answer
these questions, patients with HD, patients with alcoholic Korsakoff's syndrome, and patients with right hemisphere lesions, as well
as normal control subjects, participated in three investigations of
memory for faces and pictures. In the first and third investigations, a group of patients with presenile and senile dementia of the
Alzheimer's type (AD) was also included to provide a direct comparison of two common forms of dementia.

In the first investigation three sets of facial recognition and
matching tests were administered to 11 alcoholic Korsakoff patients,
13 patients with HD, 10 patients with AD, eight patients with localized right hemisphere lesions and 18 intact normal control subjects.
On the first test, the subjects were presented with two sets of photographs of college students. Set 1 was a 4 x 3 array of 12 photographs. The subjects were allowed to inspect the array for 45 seconds, after which the photographs were removed. Following a 90-
second delay interval, the subjects were given a 5 x 5 matrix of 25
photographs and asked to select the 12 faces that had appeared in the

original inspection set. The second test was similar to the first, but it required the subjects simply to match (rather than recognize) faces. The subjects were presented simultaneously with a 5 x 5 matrix of photographs and with a single (target) photograph of a face, and they were then asked to find the target face among the 25 comparison photographs. If the subject selected an incorrect face, he was told to continue looking until he found the correct match. This matching procedure was repeated for 12 individual target photographs.

The third test, developed by Carey and Diamond (1977), evaluated the subject's tendency to use superficial piecemeal cues (such as paraphernalia and expression), rather than more advanced configurational cues (i.e., the relationship among the eyes, nose and mouth), in their analyses of faces. On each trial of a given problem, the subject was shown a card with three photographs of unfamiliar faces, one at the top (the target face) and two at the bottom (the comparison faces). The subject was asked to indicate which of the two comparison faces was the same as the one at the top of the card. In two problem types (Types 1 and 2), paraphernalia (e.g., a hat) was used to fool the subject, and identity judgments based upon similar paraphernalia were incorrect. In two other problem types (Types 3 and 4), expression was used to fool the subject, and judgments based upon similar expressions (e.g., smiling or frowning) were incorrect. To perform consistently well on these four problem types, a subject had to rely on the configurational aspects of the faces. In addition to the four experimental problem types, there was a control problem in which neither paraphernalia nor expression were manipulated to fool the subject.

Figures 7 and 8, and Table 1 show the results for the first two tests. On the delayed recognition task (Figure 7), it is evident that all four patient groups recognized fewer of the previously presented faces than did the normal control group. Of the four patient groups, the Korsakoff and right hemisphere patients performed somewhat more poorly than did the two groups of demented patients.

The results on the face matching task (Figure 8 and Table 1) demonstrate that the patients' poor face recognition cannot be attributed entirely to a memory problem. Again, all four patient groups (especially the right hemisphere group) made many more errors (Table 1), and required more time to complete a successful match (Figure 8), than did the control group.

Figure 9 presents the findings for the Carey-Diamond test. Since few subjects made any errors on the control problem, the results for this baseline condition are not shown. On the experimental problems, all four patient groups made numerous errors due to the tendency to make identity judgments on the basis of similar paraphernalia and expression. Despite the variability among the groups on the four problem types, all of the patient groups seem to be most

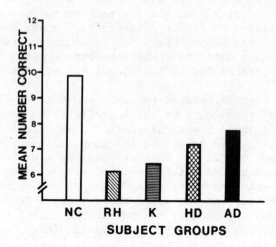

Fig. 7. Face recognition: Performance of alcoholic Korsakoffs (K),
         patients with Huntington's Disease (HD), patients with
         right hemisphere lesions (RH), patients with Alzheimer's
         Disease (AD) and normal controls (NC).

Table 1. Matching of faces: Number of S's making errors on three
          or more of the 12 trials.

Subjects	Errors (0,1,2 trials)	Errors (3 or more trials)
Normal Controls	18	0
Right Hemisphere Patients	4	4
Huntington's Disease Patients	9	4
Alzheimer's Dis- Patients	9	2
Alcoholic Korsakoff Patients	8	3

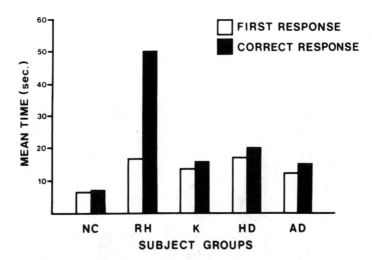

Fig. 8. Matching of faces: Performance of alcoholic Korsakoffs (K),
patients with Huntington's Disease (HD), patients with
right hemisphere lesions (RH), patients with Alzheimer's
Disease (AD) and normal controls (NC).

impaired on the paraphernalia-to-fool problems (Types 1 and 2).
These findings represent a replication of Dricker et al.'s (1978)
results with Korsakoff and right hemisphere patients, and demonstrate
that HD and AD patients are also prone to faulty stimulus analysis.
Although the normal control subjects utilized the configuration aspects of faces, the patients seemed to rely upon piecemeal, superficial features, such as paraphernalia and expression, and appeared
to ignore the configurational features of faces. If such incomplete
perceptual analysis is characteristic of these patient groups, it may
help to explain their inordinate difficulty in learning, retaining
and even perceiving nonverbal patterned materials.

     The second investigation (Biber, Butters, Rosen, Gerstman, &
Mattis, 1981), used an orientation procedure in an attempt to improve the patients' face recognition. It had been reported (Bower
& Karlin, 1974) that requiring normal subjects to make global-evaluative judgments (e.g., likeability) about a face prompts a thorough
analysis of facial features, which, in turn, results in improved
recognition. In contrast, requiring normal subjects to judge some
isolated (i.e., piecemeal) facial features (e.g., straightness of
hair) supposedly leads to a limited, inadequate analysis of facial

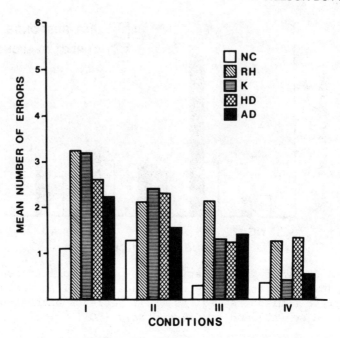

Fig. 9.   Carey Faces Test: Performance of alcoholic Korsakoffs (K),
          patients with Huntington's Disease (HD), patients with
          right hemisphere lesions (RH), patients with Alzheimer's
          Disease (AD) and normal controls (NC).

features and ultimately to poor recognition performance. Since the
groups of brain-damaged patients from our first investigation seemed
to spontaneously employ a piecemeal strategy, it was anticipated
that the introduction of global-evaluative judgments might attenuate
their severe inability to remember faces by inducing an analysis of
the configurational features of faces.

     Nine patients with alcoholic Korsakoff's syndrome, nine patients
with HD, nine patients with lesions limited to the right hemisphere,
and nine normal control subjects were administered a face recognition
task under three different levels of facial analysis. The subjects
were shown 72 photographs of male college seniors. For one set of
24 faces, the subjects were asked to judge the likeability of each
face ("high level" orientation task); for another set of 24 faces,
the subjects had to estimate the size of the person's nose ("low
level" orientation task); for the remaining 24 faces, the subjects
were asked simply to study and to try to remember the faces (free
study condition). Immediately following the presentation of the
72nd face in the study set, a forced-choice recognition test comprised of 72 trials was administered. On each trial the subjects

were shown two photographs and asked to select the one that had been exposed previously in the study set. One of the two faces had been part of the original 72 item study set; the other face was a distractor item that had not been viewed before.

The results of this study are presented in Figure 10. It is evident that the facial recognition scores of the alcoholic Korsakoff patients, but not those of the other two patient groups, improved significantly following a "high level" orientation task requiring the subjects to judge the likeability of the to-be-remembered faces. Under baseline conditions (i.e., free study), normal controls appeared spontaneously to encode faces in a manner induced by the "high level" task, whereas the Korsakoff patients employed strategies consistent with the "low level" orientation task (judgment of nose size). Thus, Korsakoff patients do not seem to process faces in a manner effective for subsequent recall or recognition unless they

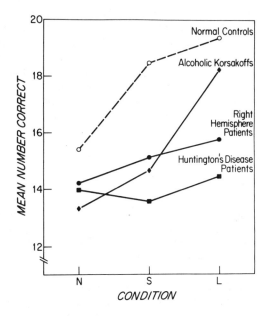

Fig. 10.   Mean number of items correctly identified on Biber et al.'s (1981) facial recognition test by each subject group. N = size-of-nose judgments; S = free study; L = Likeability judgments.

are required to carry out encoding tasks at input specifically designed to promote more complete stimulus analysis.

The results for the "high level" orientation task were consistent
with the conclusions drawn from the previously cited comparisons of
the learning and memory disorders of alcoholic Korsakoff and HD patients. These investigations showed that while both Korsakoff and
HD patients are severely impaired on various short-term memory, remote memory, and reversal learning tasks, the processes underlying
the quantitatively equivalent disorders are distinct. The present
results extend these findings to nonverbal materials. Again, the
Korsakoff patients' memory was aided by a procedure that promoted
encoding, while the impairments of the HD patients remained imperv-
ious to the same experimental manipulation. This failure of the HD
patients to improve significantly with the "high level" orientation
task, while not precluding other possible explanations, was consistent with Butters et al.'s (1979) suggestion that HD patients lack
the neuroanatomical structures necessary to consolidate and store
information.

Some mention should also be made of the differences between the
Korsakoff and the right hemisphere patients. Dricker et al. (1978)
found that these two groups performed similarly on their battery of
facial recognition, matching and encoding tasks; however, Biber et
al.'s (1981) results suggested that the perceptual impairments of
the Korsakoff and right hemisphere patients were at least quantitatively separable. Although the two patient groups' performances
were statistically indistinguishable under the free study and "low
level" conditions, the Korsakoff patients recognized more faces
than did the right hemisphere patients following the "high level"
orientation task. If, as has been reported (Carey, 1978), the
structures necessary to complete configurational analyses of faces
are located in the posterior portion of the right hemisphere, then
patients with right hemisphere lesions may fail to benefit from
"high level" orientation tasks because they lack the neuroanatomical
substrate necessary for effective configurational processing. Cor-
respondingly, despite the neuropsychological evidence that long-term
alcohol abuse affects the functions of the right hemisphere more than
those of the left (Parsons, 1975; Ryan & Butters, 1982), these critical structures within the right hemisphere appear to be relatively
intact in alcoholic Korsakoff patients and can be engaged with appropriate encoding instructions.

The third investigation comparing HD and Korsakoff patients
evaluated the beneficial effects verbal mediation and labeling might
have on the amnesic and demented patients' ability to remember pictorial materials. In the other studies reviewed in this section,
it was found that manipulations of experimental variables such as
rehearsal time, intertrial rest intervals and orientation instructions resulted in improved performance only for the alcoholic Korsa-

Korsakoff patients. However, since HD is a progressive dementia in
which language abilities remain relatively intact until the terminal
stages of the disease (Butters et al., 1978), the possibility remained that providing these patients with verbal labels and mediators
might reduce their severe difficulties in remembering pictorial stimuli. In view of numerous reports that alcoholic Korsakoff patients
do not encode all of the semantic attributes of verbal material, there
is reason to believe that verbal mediators would have little impact on
their memory problems. Likewise, the very prevalent and severe language impairments that usually accompany AD (Miller, 1977) could eliminate any beneficial consequences verbal mediators might have on the
Alzheimer patients' ability to remember pictorial materials.

        In this study, Shneidman's (1952) Make-A-Picture Story Test
(MAPS) was modified to assess the pictorial memory of 14 HD patients,
11 alcoholic Korsakoff patients, 8 patients with lesions restricted
to the right hemisphere, 12 patients with AD and 18 normal control
subjects. Two conditions were employed: a no-story followed by a
story. On the no-story condition, the subjects were shown pictures
of six backgrounds (e.g., a raft floating on a large body of water,
a living room) on which three cut-out human or animal figures had
been placed. For example, a superman figure, a figure of an angry
man and a figure of a happy little boy were placed in the living room
scene. The subjects were instructed to remember the identity and location of the specific figures on each scene and were allowed 30 seconds to study each of the six scenes. Five minutes following the
presentation of the sixth scene the subjects were administered a forced-choice recognition test consisting of 15 pairs of figures. The
subjects were required to indicate for each pair which of the two cut
out figures they had seen in one of the previously exposed scenes.
For all 15 pairs, one of the figures had been exposed previously, and
the other was a distractor item not previously seen by the subjects.

        Ten minutes after the recognition test, a recall test was admin-
istered. The 6 backgrounds were placed, one at a time, in front of
the subjects and 33 cut-out figures (18 targets, 15 distractors) were
distributed symmetrically around the background. The subjects were
asked to select from the 33 figures the ones that had been associated
with the scene during the original exposure (learning) trial. The
examiner recorded the identity of the figures selected, location of
the figures' positions, and the figures' spatial orientations.

        After a 15-minute rest interval, the story condition was admin-
istered. Six different background scenes, each with three new cut-
out figures, were shown to the subjects. The major difference in
procedure was that during the 30-second study period provided for
each picture, the subjects were read a story about the events trans-
piring in the stimulus scene. Each story related not only what was
occurring in the scene, but also what had led to the depicted situation and how the situation would be resolved in the immediate future.

As in the no-story condition, recognition and recall tests followed
the presentation of the sixth background.

The groups' performance on the recognition tests are shown in
Figure 11. Although in both story and no-story conditions the patients correctly recognized slightly fewer figures than the normal control subjects, their performance was considerably better than change
(7.5 correct). Thus, it appeared that amnesic and demented patients
could accurately discriminate familiar from unfamiliar figures.

Despite the patients' relatively intact recognition performance,
their recall of figures, as seen in Figure 12, was severely impaired.
A two-way analysis of variance yielded highly significant group, condition (story vs. no-story), and interaction (group x condition) effects. On the no-story condition, all four patient groups recalled
significantly fewer figures than did the normal control group. Of
the four patient groups, the alcoholic Korsakoff and the AD patients
were the most impaired, although there was considerable variability
within each patient group in terms of degree of impairment.

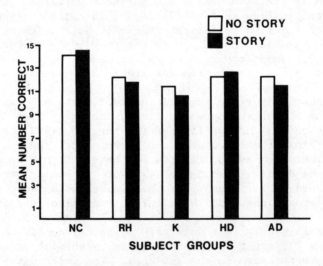

Fig. 11.   Recognition performance on the picture memory (MAPS) test
           under the story and no-story conditions. K = alcoholic
           Korsakoffs; HD = patients with Huntington's Disease; RH =
           patients with right hemisphere lesions; AD = patients with
           Alzheimer's Disease; NC = normal controls.

The results for the story condition (Figure 12) clearly show
that the four patient groups were aided differentially by the presentation of verbal mediators. The recall scores of the HD and the
right hemisphere patients were significantly improved by the recitation of the story, while the recall scores of the Korsakoff and
AD patients appeared insensitive to this mnemonic aid. It is important to note that the improvement of the HD and right hemisphere
patients was not due to their slightly superior performance on the
no-story condition. When the amount of improvement between the
story and no-story conditions was analyzed with a covariance design
which statistically corrected for performance on the no-story condition, the HD and right hemisphere patients continued to demonstrate
significantly more improvement than did the other two patient groups.
Furthermore, no significant correlation was found between performance
on the no-story condition and the amount of improvement induced by
the story.

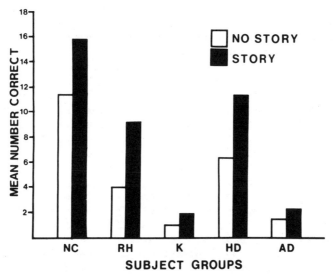

Figure 12.   Recall (correct figures in correct location) performance
              on the picture memory (MAPS) test under the story and
              no-story conditions. K = alcoholic Korsakoffs; HD =
              patients with Huntington's Disease; RH = patients with
              right hemisphere lesions; AD = patients with Alzheimer's
              Disease; NC = normal controls.

The findings of this last investigation, especially those relating to the HD and Korsakoff patients, are of special importance
because they provide additional legitimacy for other dissociations
noted in this section of the chapter. Although the studies of the
patients' short-term memory, retrograde amnesia, and memory for
faces suggested significant differences between HD and Korsakoff
patients, none of them provided the elusive double dissociation
needed to firmly establish our claim of qualitative differences in
the memory disorders of the two groups. The fact that the Korsakoff, but not the HD, patients were affected by rehearsal time, intertrial rest intervals, and orientation procedures, might have been
a reflection of the totally debilitating effects of dementia, rather
than an indicator of qualitative differences in information processing. However, in the present study, the double dissociation between
groups and tasks has been completed. For the first time in our comparative studies of Korsakoff and HD patients, an experimental manipulation (i.e., the introduction of verbal mediators) enhanced the
learning performance of the HD patients more than that of the Korsakoff patients. As anticipated on the basis of their lack of aphasic symptoms, the HD patients were able to utilize language cues to
facilitate associations between the cut-out figures and specific
scenes and thereby improve their contextual memory. Conversely, the
alcoholic Korsakoff patients, who are reputed to have deficits in
verbal encoding (Butters & Cermak, 1980), were unable to utilize the
stories in such a beneficial manner. It has been reported by Winokur
and Kinsbourne (1978), that the contextual memory of alcoholic Korsakoff patients can be improved by increasing the saliency of cues
present in the learning environment, but none of the procedures employed by these investigators involved the introduction of verbal
mediators.

Although the present findings may support the thesis that HD
and alcoholic Korsakoff patients have qualitatively distinct memory
deficits, they offer little help in specifying the exact nature of
the cognitive disorders. Clearly, our previous suggestion that HD
patients lack the neuroanatomical structures necessary for storing
information is untenable in light of this last memory study. If
the HD patients had a storage problem, the introduction of verbal
mediators should have been as unsuccessful as Biber et al.'s (1981)
orientation task and Butters et al.'s (1979) use of increased rehearsal times and intertrial rest intervals. An alternative explanation has been offered by Weingartner, Caine and Ebert (1979), who
have suggested that HD patients' verbal memory deficits may be due
to underlying deficiencies in the encoding process. In view of the
present results, this hypothesis may have merit; however, it will
be necessary to elucidate how these encoding impairments differ from
those that seem to characterize the performance of alcoholic Korsakoff patients.

Like the HD patients, the patients with right hemisphere lesions also benefited significantly from the introduction of the verbal mediators. The recitation of the stories apparently prompted a more complete analysis of the elements of the pictures and may also have provided valuable cues for linking the figures with specific contexts. Although there has been abundant documentation of the severe visuoperceptive deficits which accompany right hemisphere damage (Milner, 1971; Benton, 1979), the feasibility of employing the linguistic capacities of the intact left hemisphere in rehabilitative efforts has not received adequate attention. Boller and DeRenzi (1967) have reported that right hemisphere patients, as well as patients with left hemisphere lesions and intact control subjects, find it easier to form associations between meaningful (i.e., verbalizable) than between meaningless (i.e., nonverbalizable) figures, but they did not evaluate whether their two patient groups would be differentially affected by imposing explicit verbal lables on the figures. The present findings suggest that it may be worthwhile to explore both the rehabilitative limits of verbal mediators and the mechanisms by which language can alter the perceptual and memory disorders of patients with right hemisphere lesions.

The similarities and differences in the memory impairments of the HD and the AD patients should not go unnoticed. The findings of the previously reported face recognition, and the matching and encoding tasks might have given credence to the notion that demented patients, regardless of etiology, are essentially identical in terms of their cognitive dysfunctions. It is evident, however, from the picture memory study, that the dementias (like the amnesias) should not be treated as a single disorder. While the HD patients can utilize language as a mnemonic for circumventing their pictorial memory problems, patients with Alzheimer's Disease have lost this opportunity to employ linguistic mnemonics due to the aphasic symptoms apparent early in the disease process. The relevance of this difference for the demented patients' ability to remain in a non-institutionalized setting should not escape an audience sophisticated in neuropsychology.

In summary, the results of these comparative studies of HD and Korsakoff patients reinforce our previous conclusions based upon a scrutiny of various forms of amnesia. These recent investigations of facial and pictorial memory, as well as the studies concerned with verbal learning, remote memory and discrimination learning, suggest that HD, Korsakoff and even AD patients fail to acquire and retrieve information for quite different reasons. The fact that all of the amnesic and demented groups discussed in this paper had low MQ's revealed little about the nature of their impairments. Thus, reliance on a single quantitative measure of memory (e.g, the MQ) for the assessment of amnesic symptoms, may have as many limitations as does the utilization of an isolated score on a naming or fluency test for the full description of aphasia.

REFERENCES

Albert, M.S., Butters, N., & Brandt, J.   Memory for remote events in
    alcoholics. Journal of Studies on Alcohol, 1980, 41, 1071–1081.
Albert, M.S., Butters, N. & Brandt, J.   Patterns of remote memory in
    amnesic and demented patients. Archives of Neurology, 1981a,
    38, 495–500.
Albert, M.S., Butters, N., & Brandt, J.   Development of remote memory
    loss in patients with Huntington's Disease. Journal of Clinical
    Neuropsychology, 1981b, 3, 1–12.
Albert, M.S., Butters, N., & Levin, J.   Temporal gradients in the
    retrograde amnesia of patients with alcoholic Korsakoff's dis-
    ease. Archives of Neurology, 1979, 36, 211–216.
Baddeley, A.D., & Warrington, E.K.   Amnesia and the distinction be-
    tween long- and short-term memory. Journal of Verbal Learning
    and Verbal Behavior, 1970, 9, 176–189.
Benson, D., & Geschwind, N.   Shrinking retrograde amnesia. Journal
    of Neurology, Neurosurgery, and Psychiatry, 1967, 30, 539–544.
Benton, A.   Visuoperceptive, visuospatial, and visuoconstructive dis-
    orders. In K.M. Heilman & E. Valenstein (Eds.), Clinical neuro-
    psychology. New York: Oxford University Press, 1979.
Biber, C., Butters, N., Rosen, J., Gerstman, L., & Mattis, S.   Encod-
    ing strategies and recognition of faces by alcoholic Korsakoff
    and other brain-damaged patients. Journal of Clinical Neuropsy-
    chology, 1981, 3, 315–330.
Boller, F., & DeRenzi, E.   Relationship between visual memory defects
    and hemispheric locus of lesion. Neurology, 1967, 17, 1052–1058.
Bower, G.H., & Karlin, M.B.   Depth of processing pictures of faces and
    recognition memory. Journal of Experimental Psychology, 1974,
    103, 751–757.
Butters, N.   Amnesic disorders. In K.M. Heilman & E. Valenstein
    (Eds.), Clinical neuropsychology. New York: Oxford University
    Press, 1979.
Butters, N., & Albert, M.S.   Processes underlying failures to recall
    remote events. In L.S. Cermak (Ed.), Human memory and amnesia.
    Hillsdale, N.J.: Lawrence Erlbaum Associates, 1982.
Butters, N., Albert, M.S., & Sax, D.   Investigations of the memory
    disorders of patients with Huntington's Disease. In T. Chase,
    N. Wexler & A. Barbeau (Eds.), Advances in neurology, volume
    23: Huntington's disease. New York: Raven Press, 1979.
Butters, N., & Cermak, L.S.   Some analyses of amnesic syndromes in
    brain damaged patients. In R. Isaacson & K. Pribram (Eds.), The
    hippocampus, volume 2. New York: Plenum Press, 1975.
Butters, N., & Cermak, L.S. (Eds.) Alcoholic Korsakoff's Syndrome:
    An information-processing approach to amnesia. New York: Aca-
    demic Press, 1980.
Butters, N., & Grady, M.   Effect of predistractor delays on the
    short-term memory performance of patients with Korsakoff's and
    Huntington's Disease. Neuropsychologia, 1977, 13, 701–705.
Butters, N., Sax, D., Montgomery, K., & Tarlow, S.   Comparison of the

neuropsychological deficits associated with early and advanced Huntington's Disease. Archives of Neurology, 1978, 35. 585-589.

Butters, N., Tarlow, S., Cermak, L.S., & Sax, D. A comparison of the information processing deficits of patients with Huntington's Chorea and Korsakoff's Syndrome. Cortex, 1976, 12, 134-144.

Caine, E.D., Ebert, M.H., & Weingartner, H. An outline for the analysis of dementia: The memory disorder of Huntington's Disease. Neurology, 1977, 27, 1087-1092.

Carey, S. A case study: Face recognition. In E.C.T. Walker (Ed.), Explorations in the biology of language. Vermont: Bradford Books, 1978.

Carey, S., & Diamond, R. From piecemeal to configurational representation of faces. Science, 1977, 195, 312-314.

Carlen, P.L., Wilkinson, D.A., Wortzman, G., Holgate, R., Cordingley, J., Lee, M.A., Huzar, L., Moddel, G., Singh, R., Kiraly, L., & Rankin, J.G. Cerebral atrophy and functional deficits in alcoholics without clinically apparent liver disease. Neurology, 1981, 31, 377-385.

Cermak, L.S. The encoding capacity of a patient with amnesia due to encephalitis. Neuropsychologia, 1976, 14, 311-326.

Cohen, N.J., & Squire, L.R. Retrograde amnesia and remote memory impairment. Neuropsychologia, 1981, 19, 337-356.

Drachman, D.A., & Adams, R.D. Herpes simplex and acute inclusion body encephalitis. Archives of Neurology, 1962, 7, 45-63.

Drachman, D.A., & Arbit, J. Memory and the hippocampal complex. Archives of Neurology, 1966, 15, 52-61.

Dricker, J., Butters, N., Berman, G., Samuels, I., & Carey, S. Recognition and encoding of faces by alcoholic Korsakoff and right hemisphere patients. Neuropsychologia, 1978, 16, 683-695.

Fedio, P., & Van-Buren, J. Memory deficits during electrical stimulation of the speech cortex in conscious man. Brain and Language, 1974, 1, 29-42.

Goldberg, E., Antin, S.P., Bilder, R.M., Jr., Hughes, J.E.O., & Mattis, S. Retrograde amnesia: Possible role of mesencephalic reticular activation in long-term memory. Science, 1981, 213, 1392-1394.

Huppert, F.A., & Piercy, M. Recognition memory in amnesic patients: A defect of acquisition? Neuropsychologia, 1977, 15, 643-652.

Huppert, F.A., & Piercey, M. Dissociation between learning and remembering in organic amnesia. Nature, 1978, 275, 317-318.

Huppert, F.A., & Piercy, M. Normal and abnormal forgetting in organic amnesia: Effect of locus of lesion. Cortex, 1979, 15, 385-390.

Lhermitte, F., & Signoret, J.L. Neurological analysis and differentiation of amnesic syndromes. Revue Neurologique, 1972, 126, 161-178.

Lindqvist, G., & Norlen, G. Korsakoff's Syndrome after operation on ruptured aneurysm of the anterior communicating artery. Acta Psychiatrica Scandinavica, 1966, 42, 24-34.

Lishman, W.A. Cerebral disorder in alcoholism: Syndromes of impair-
    ment. Brain, 1981, 104, 1-20.
Meudell, P., Butters, N., & Montgomery, K. Role of rehearsal in the
    short-term memory performance of patients with Korsakoff's and
    Huntington's Disease. Neuropsychologia, 1978, 16, 507-510.
Miller, E. Abnormal aging: The psychology of senile and presenile
    dementia. London: Wiley, 1977.
Milner, B. Amnesia following operation on the temporal lobes. In
    C.W.M. Whitty & O.L. Zangwill (Eds.), Amnesia. London: Butters-
    worth, 1966.
Milner, B. Memory and the medial temporal regions of the brain. In
    K.H. Pribram & D.E. Broadbent (Eds.), Biology of memory. New
    York: Academic Press, 1970.
Milner, B. Interhemispheric differences in the localization of psy-
    chological processes in man. British Medical Bulletin, 1971,
    27, 272-275.
Oscar-Berman, M., & Zola-Morgan, S.M. Comparative neuropsychology
    and Korsakoff's Syndrome. I-Spatial and visual reversal learn-
    ing. Neuropsychologia, 1980a, 18, 499-512.
Oscar-Berman, M., & Zola-Morgan, S.M. Comparative neuropsychology
    and Korsakoff's Syndrome. II - Two-choice visual discrimina-
    tion learning. Neuropsychologia, 1980b, 18, 513-525.
Parsons, O.A. Brain damage in alcoholics: Altered states of uncon-
    sciousness. In M. Gross (Ed.), Alcohol intoxication and with-
    drawal II. New York: Plenum Press, 1975.
Peterson, L.R., & Peterson, M.J. Short-term retention of individual
    verbal items. Journal of Experimental Psychology, 1959, 58,
    193-198.
Ryan, C., & Butters, N. Evidence for a continuum-of-impairment en-
    compassing male alcoholic Korsakoff patients and chronic alco-
    holic men. Alcoholism: Clinical and Experimental Research,
    1980, 4, 190-198.
Ryan, C., & Butters, N. Cognitive deficits in alcoholics. In B.
    Kissin & H. Begleiter (Eds.), Biology of alcoholism, volume 6.
    Biological pathogenesis of alcoholism. New York: Plenum Press,
    1982.
Samuels, I., Butters, N., & Fedio, P. Short-term memory disorders
    following temporal lobe removals in humans. Cortex, 1972, 8,
    283-298.
Samuels, I., Butters, N., & Goodglass, H. Visual memory deficits
    following cortical and limbic lesions: Effect of field present-
    ation. Physiology and Behavior, 1971, 6, 447-452.
Samuels, I., Butters, N., Goodglass, H., & Brody, B. A comparison
    of subcortical and cortical damage on short-term visual and
    auditory memory. Neuropsychologia, 1971, 9, 293-306.
Schneidman, E.S. Make a picture story test. New York: The Psycho-
    ological Corporation, 1952.
Scoville, W.B., & Milner, B. Loss of recent memory after bilateral
    hippocampal lesions. Journal of Neurology, Neurosurgery, and
    Psychiatry, 1957, 20, 11-21.

Shallice, T., & Warrington, E.K. The independent functioning of
    verbal memory stores: A neuropsychological study. Quarterly
    Journal of Experimental Psychology, 1970, 22, 261-273.
Squire, L.R. Two forms of human amnesia: An analysis of forgetting.
    The Journal of Neuroscience, 1981, 1, 635-640.
Squire, L.R., & Cohen, N.J. Remote memory, retrograde amnesia, and
    the neuropsychology of memory. In L.S. Cermak (Ed.), Human
    memory and amnesia. Hillsdale, N.J.: Lawrence Erlbaum Assoc-
    iates, 1982.
Squire, L.R., & Moore, R.Y. Dorsal thalamic lesions in a noted case
    of chronic memory dysfunction. Annals of Neurology, 1979, 6,
    503-506.
Squire, L.R., & Slater, P.C. Anterograde and retrograde memory im-
    pairment in chronic amnesia. Neuropsychologia, 1978, 16, 312-
    322.
Teuber, H.L., Milner, B., & Vaughan, H. Persistent anterograde am-
    nesia after stab wound of the basal brain. Neuropsychologia,
    1968, 6, 267-282.
Victor, M., Adams, R.D., & Collins, G.H. The Wernicke-Korsakoff Syn-
    drome. Philadelphia: F.A. Davis, 1971.
Warrington, E.K. The double dissociation of short- and long-term
    memory deficits. In L.S. Cermak (Ed.), Human memory and amnesia.
    Hillsdale, N.J.: Lawrence Erlbaum Associates, 1981.
Warrington, E.K., Logue, V., & Pratt, R.T.C. The anatomical local-
    ization of selective impairment of auditory verbal short-term
    memory. Neuropsychologia, 1972, 9, 377-387.
Warrington, E.K., & Shallice, T. The selective impairment of audi-
    tory verbal short-term memory. Brain, 1969, 92, 885-896.
Warrington, E.K., & Shallice, T. Neuropsychological evidence of
    visual storage in short-term memory tasks. Quarterly Journal
    of Experimental Psychology, 1972, 24, 30-40.
Warrington, E.K., & Weiskrantz, L. An analysis of short-term and
    long-term memory defects in man. In J.A. Deutsch (Ed.), The
    physiological basis of memory. New York: Academic Press, 1973.
Weingartner, H., Caine, E., & Ebert, M.H. Imagery, encoding, and
    retrieval of information from memory: Some specific encoding-
    retrieval changes in Huntington's Disease. Journal of Abnormal
    Psychology, 1979, 88, 52-58.
Wilson, R.S., Kaszniak, A.W., & Fox, J.H. Remote memory in senile
    dementia. Cortex, 1981, 17, 41-48.
Winokur, G., & Kinsbourne, M. Contextual cueing as an aid to Korsa-
    koff amnesics. Neuropsychologia, 1978, 16, 671-682.

RECOVERY OF FUNCTION FOLLOWING BRAIN DAMAGE: HOMEOSTASIS AT

DOPAMINERGIC SYNAPSES

Edward M. Stricker and Michael J. Zigmond

Departments of Biological Sciences, Psychology, and
Psychiatry
University of Pittsburgh
Pittsburgh, PA 15260

INTRODUCTION

Damage to the central nervous system is often accompanied by
frank behavioral symptoms. Although the damaged neurons do not regenerate, nevertheless in most cases there will be some recovery
of function, the extent of which will depend on the size and location of the damage, the function in question, and the time since
the cerebral accident or injury. Some of this recovery might be
attributed to reversal of certain secondary effects of the damage,
such as hemorrhage and edema. However, there are cases in which
those processes do not appear to be responsible for the recovery
of function that is observed. For the past decade we have been in-
vestigating such a case and exploring its neurochemical bases.

Our studies have involved rats with experimental lesions of
the dopamine-containing neurons that project to the forebrain from
cell bodies in the mesencephalon. Following specific lesions that
destroy 90-95 percent or more of these neurons, animals eat and
drink nothing, even when surrounded by food and fluids that are
both familiar and palatable. Consequently, they steadily lose
weight and ultimately starve to death unless the experimenter in-
tervenes and initiates a program of forced alimentation. After
periods of such tube feeding that may extend to weeks or even to
months, the brain-damaged animals gradually begin to eat and drink
voluntarily and maintain their body weight without assistance. Yet
when they are killed and their brains are examined months after the
lesions were made, biochemical analyses reveal that dopamine (DA)
depletions still exceed 90-95 percent. If the initial dysfunction
resulted from damage to the dopaminergic neurons, what accounts for
the observed recovery of function?

161

We believe that the answer to this paradox lies in the adaptive ability of residual elements of the dopaminergic system to compensate for the damage, and that this plasticity in the central nervous system has considerable significance for our understanding of brain function and disease. In considering these issues, we have divided our essay into three parts. First, we will briefly describe the behavioral syndrome which results from extensive damage to the central dopaminergic neurons in rats. Next, we will identify some of the neurochemical changes resulting from such brain damage that appear to contribute to the observed recovery of function. Finally, we will consider several implications of this analysis, both for the general issue of homeostasis at catecholaminergic synapses, and for the specific neurological disorders of Parkinsonism and Minimal Brain Dysfunction.

Behavioral Syndrome

The behavioral syndrome includes the initial loss of eating and drinking after the brain damage, the gradual recovery of function which normally occurs when animals are maintained by intragastric intubation of nutrients, and the residual deficits which remain. The syndrome was first observed and characterized in rats with bilateral damage to the lateral hypothalamus and was, therefore, attributed to the destruction of specific feeding and drinking centers in the hypothalamus (Anand & Brobeck, 1951; Teitelbaum & Epstein, 1962). However, with the discovery that monoaminergic neurons traverse the ventral diencephalon (Anden, Dahlstrom, Fuxe, Larsson, Olson, & Ungerstedt, 1966; Moore, Bhatnagar & Heller, 1971), the issue arose as to whether the syndrome resulted from destruction of hypothalamic tissue per se or interruption of the fibers of passage (Ungerstedt, 1971; Oltmans & Harvey, 1972; Fibiger, Zis, & McGeer, 1973; Zigmond & Stricker, 1972, 1973).

Its resolution required the use of three new techniques which had been developed for creating specific destruction of brain neurons. Each involves the intracerebral injection of a synthetic analogue of a natural neurotransmitter. The first neurotoxin used was 6-hydroxydopamine (6-HDA), a structural analogue of DA and norepinephrine (NE) which depletes the brain of these catecholamines whether administered directly into brain tissue or via the cerebroventricular system. Although this drug readily oxidizes to yield such cytotoxic compounds as hydrogen peroxide and quinones, it is selectively transported into catecholaminergic terminals. Consequently, it usually is possible to limit most of the damage primarily to those cells (e.g., Hedreen & Chalmers, 1972). The other chemical treatments involve intracerebral injections of 5,7-dihydroxytryptamine, an analogue of serotonin that can be used to destroy serotonergic neurons (Bjorklund, Baumgarten, & Rensch, 1975), and kainic acid, an analogue of glutamic acid that apparently destroys cell bodies in the brain without damaging fibers of passage (McGeer & McGeer, 1976; Schwarcz & Coyle, 1977). Neither serotonin-depleting brain lesions nor administration of kainic acid into the lateral hypothalamus was found to produce aphagia and adipsia (Saller & Stricker, 1978; Stricker, Swerdloff, & Zigmond, 1978; Peterson & Moore, 1980). However, administration of 6-HDA was effective in this regard, whenever DA depletions exceeded 90-95 percent (Ungerstedt, 1971; Zigmond & Stricker, 1972). These results were obtained even when animals were pretreated with drugs that prevented uptake of 6-HDA into noradrenergic nerve terminals and thereby limited its neurotoxic effects to the dopaminergic neurons (Stricker & Zigmond, 1974).

Rats with large DA-depleting brain lesions are now known to have debilitating sensorimotor disturbances, such as akinesia, catalepsy, and impaired orientation to stimuli (Marshall & Teitelbaum, 1974; Marshall, Levitan, & Stricker, 1976). Consequently, the same lesions that abolish feeding and drinking also eliminate other motivational activities, such as sexual, thermoregulatory and punishment-avoidance behaviors (Cooper, Breese, Howard, & Grant, 1972; Caggiula, Shaw, Antelman, & Edwards, 1976; Van Zoeren & Stricker, 1977). Their aphagia and adipsia, therefore, appears not to reflect specific problems in ingestive behavior, but more fundamental problems of responding to interoceptive and exteroceptive stimulation. This might occur if sensory signals normally increased neural firing in dopaminergic neurons (Nieoullon, Cheramy, & Glowinski, 1977; Chiodo, Antelman, Caggiula, & Lineberry, 1980), since it should then take a more intense stimulus to promote behavioral activation in lesioned animals than in controls. These considerations are consistent with findings that brain-damaged rats show normal motor activity and exploratory behavior when placed in a shallow ice bath, and swim normally when placed in a large tank of tepid water (Levitt & Teitelbaum, 1975; Marshall et al., 1976). They also move and respond appropriately when placed among a colony of kittens. These potentially life-threatening situations are not the only ones that produce reliable and dramatic improvements of sensorimotor functions; for example, male rats that are cataleptic and akinetic nevertheless pursue and copulate successfully with estrogen-progesterone-treated female rats (Caggiula et al., 1976). In each case, a higher level of arousal appears to be required for brain-damaged animals to initiate the appropriate behavior.

In order to assess the sensorimotor skills of brain-damaged rats more quantitatively, a series of nine neurological examinations was developed and a rating scale used to grade each rat (Marshall & Teitelbaum, 1974; Marshall et al., 1976). Animals were found to be akinetic and cataleptic soon after the lesions, and did not orient well to touch of the body sides. Yet, they did show some sensorimotor capability. For example, they usually could turn around when placed on an inclined plane and orient appropriately when their forepaws were pinched. These impairments generally abated in parallel with the gradual recovery of ingestive behavior. The tests in which the animals initially had their poorest performance were the ones that would be expected to provide the least amount of activation. Thus, their recovery can be interpreted as an improved capacity to become activated by relatively low levels of stimulation. Similarly, the distinct stages identified in the recovery from aphagia and adipsia, which were first identified in animals with lateral hypothalamic lesions (Teitelbaum & Epstein, 1962), each reflect a reduction of the extra stimulation required to promote ingestion. For example, lesioned rats that do not at first eat or drink anything (Stage I) later become willing to consume foods that provide the activating influence of high palatability (Stage II), especially if the animals are also given amphetamine or other nonspecific activators (Antelman, Rowland, & Fisher, 1976; Zigmond, Heffner, & Stricker, 1980). Still later, animals accept dry laboratory chow, but do not drink unless the water is sweetened with sucrose or saccharin (Stage III), and ultimately, they again maintain body weight by eating chow and drinking tap water (Stage IV).

Even after apparent recovery of function, rats with large DA-depleting brain lesions have behavioral deficits. For example, unlike control rats, they do not eat following treatments that abruptly decrease glucose utilization or drink during acute hypovolemia (Epstein & Teitelbaum, 1967; Stricker & Wolf, 1967). These impairments appear to be no more specific than the initial aphagia and adipsia, since the brain-damaged rats not only fail to eat and drink but also become akinetic and cataleptic (Stricker, Cooper, Marshall, & Zigmond, 1979; Snyder, Stricker, & Zigmond, 1980). It is shown in Figure 1 that such a regression to an earlier stage of recovery seems to be most likely when the brain damage is extensive and the regulatory imbalance is particularly large. In contrast, the lesioned animals increase their food and water intake appropriately when the treatments are more moderate and long-lasting (Stricker, Friedman, & Zigmond, 1975; Stricker, 1976). When the treatments are too mild, however, behavioral deficits again are observed, but not in association with detectable sensorimotor impairments; hence, they probably result from a continued insensitivity of the brain-damaged rats to relatively weak stimuli. As would be expected from this analysis, male rats with DA-depleting brain lesions show a greater dependence on the sexual eliciting properties of the female for the initiation and maintenance of copulatory behavior than control rats do (Cagiula et al., 1976). Similarly, they show permanent reductions in the level at which body weight is maintained (Powley & Keesey, 1970; Stricker & Zigmond, 1974), presumably because it takes a greater stimulus of hunger to provoke feeding in them and less food intake to cause that stimulus to slip below threshold levels of activation.

These findings suggest that the range of stimuli which elicit

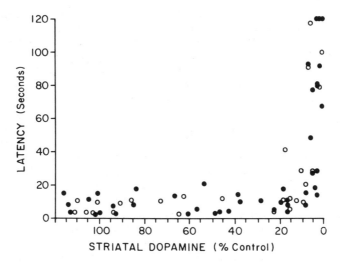

Fig. 1. Latency of rats to move all four limbs when placed on a
         table, as a function of striatal dopamine depletions pro-
         duced by intraventricular (●) or intracisternal 6-hydroxy-
         dopamine treatments (○). This test for akinesia was con-
         ducted 30 min and 120 min after rats had been given 500 mg/kg
         2-deoxyglucose. Each symbol represents the averaged value
         from the two tests for a different animal. (Snyder et al.,
         1980).

motivated behaviors is severely contracted by DA-depleting brain lesions. With recovery of function, this range gradually widens and
rats become more responsive to weak stimuli and less intolerant of
strong challenges, although residual deficits indicate that recovery
is not complete even when animals again are consuming food and water.
At any given postoperative time, an animal's ability to respond to a
particular type of stimulus thus appears to be a function of its stage
of recovery, the intensity of the stimulus, and the nature of the
testing conditions.

Biochemical Changes

    One possible explanation for the recovery of function after DA-
depleting brain lesions is that the residual dopaminergic neurons
gradually assume the functions of the entire pathway (Zigmond &
Stricker, 1974; Stricker & Zigmond, 1976). In support of this hypothesis, we find that aphagia, adipsia, and the general sensorimotor
dysfunctions are reinstated in animals recovered from the initial effects of their brain lesions when central dopaminergic neurons are
further disrupted by an additional 6-HDA treatment or by administration of either α-methyl-p-tyrosine (which inhibits catecholamine

synthesis) or spiroperidol (which blocks DA receptors) (Heffner, Zigmond, & Stricker, 1977; Marshall, 1979). Conversely, anorexic brain-
damaged animals begin to eat after administration of apomorphine
(which stimulates DA receptors) (Ljungberg & Ungerstedt, 1976).
These results would not be expected if resumption of feeding results
from transfer of functions formerly served by DA-containing neurons
to another neurochemical pathway.

There is accumulating evidence that DA (and NE) activity is reg-
ulated at the synaptic level. For example, there are compensatory
increases in release and synthesis of DA and in the number of DA receptors in the central nervous system following the administration of
receptor antagonists (Westerink, 1979; Seeman, 1980). Receptor activity also is reduced by damage to dopaminergic pathways, since there
are fewer neurons releasing DA. If receptors are activated by DA
from many adjacent pathways, and if communication within individual
neurons is equivalent, then one of the bases for recovery of function
following subtotal damage to DA-containing neurons may be provided by
increases in the synthesis and release of DA in residual dopaminergic
neurons, together with a reduced inactivation of DA by reuptake into
axon terminals (due to their diminished number) and an increased effect of DA at postsynaptic neurons.

Four lines of evidence support this concept of recovery. First,
changes in the levels of DA metabolites are less marked than the reduction in DA levels that is produced by intraventricular 6-HDA treatments. For example, we find that the loss of 74 percent of striatal
DA is accompanied by only a 45 percent decline in dihydroxyphenylacetic acid (DOPAC), one of the principal metabolites of DA. This is illustrated in Table 1. In fact, as can be seen in Figure 2, for DA depletions above 50%, the ratio of DOPAC to DA rises steadily with increasing lesion size. If one takes DA content to reflect the number

Table 1.   Effect of 6-HDA on Dopamine, Dihydroxyphenylacetic Acid,
           and Tyrosine Hydroxylase Activity in Striatum

	Control	6-HDA	% Control
DA (ug/g)	7.00 ± .33	1.55 ± .50	22.1
DOPAC (ug/g)	2.78 ± .39	1.52 ± .12	54.7
TH (nmoles/mg/min)	.950 ± .023	.474 ± .046	49.9

Note: Rats were given 250 ug 6-HDA 21 days prior to sacrifice. Tyrosine hydroxylase was measured at pH 5.6 (pH optimum for this area)
and in the presence of a saturating concentration of cofactor.
Values represent the means ± S.E.M. for groups of four. Data from
Acheson et al., 1979.

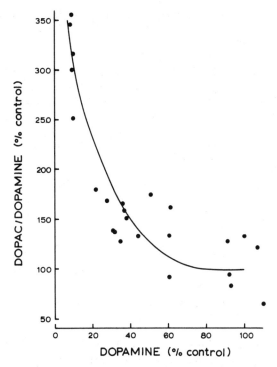

Fig. 2.   DOPAC concentration in striatum as a function of DA depletion.
          Animals given 6-HDA were sacrificed 3-21 days later, and the DOPAC
          and DA content of striatum determined. Since DA content ap-
          pears to be an index of the number of residual terminals
          (e.g., it correlated with the number of high-affinity DA up-
          take sites) results are expressed as a ratio of DOPAC/DA. An
          increase in this ratio may indicate an increase in amount of
          DOPAC formed per residual terminal (Acheson et al., 1979).

of residual dopaminergic terminals, an increase in DA turnover in
these residual neurons is suggested (Acheson et al., 1979). This hypothesis is consistent with the relative increases in the production
of homovanillic acid (another metabolite of DA), in the synthesis of
DA following subtotal destruction of dopaminergic neurons (Agid et
al., 1973; Hefti et al., 1980) and with the increased sensitivity of
rats with DA-depleting brain lesions to the effects of α-methyl-p-
tyrosine on food intake and sensorimotor function (Zigmond & Stricker,
1973; Marshall, 1979; Stricker et al., 1979).

Second, as with the DOPAC content, the effect of 6-HDA on the
striatal activity of tyrosine hydroxylase, the rate limiting enzyme
in the biosynthesis of DA (and NE), is less severe than is the decline
in DA. This can also be seen in Table 1. This apparent increase in

enzyme activity in residual nerve terminals has been well-studied in
the noradrenergic projection from locus coeruleus to hippocampus and
appears to result from two temporally distinct processes (Acheson et
al., 1980; Acheson & Zigmond, 1981). At first, within 36 hours after
the lesion, the elevation in enzyme activity results from activation
of existing enzyme molecules. Subsequently, this activation is gradually replaced by an increase in the amount of enzyme in the residual
terminals. Such changes in tyrosine hydroxylase activity have also
been produced by catecholamine receptor antagonists and by reserpine
(which depletes the nerve terminals of catecholamines) (Zivkovic et
al., 1974; Reis et al., 1975).

The decrease in DA uptake represents another adaptive change.
This change, which was closely correlated with the decrease in DA
content of tissues, does not appear to be an active response to the
lesion, but simply results from the loss of DA terminals and their
high-affinity transport sites (Zigmond & Stricker, 1980). Nevertheless, it may serve an important function. Although it is likely that
DA released from one terminal does not normally gain access to receptors which are in the proximity of other terminals, a decrease in the
number of uptake sites following 6-HDA treatment should also decrease
the rate at which transmitter diffusing from residual terminals is
inactivated, and thereby permit it to act on more distant target
cells. This hormone-like action would be analogous to the restora-
tive effects of adrenomedullary catecholamines after destruction of
peripheral noradrenergic neurons (Cannon & Rosenblueth, 1949).

Finally, destruction of DA (and NE) terminals by 6-HDA is followed by an apparent increase in the number of postsynaptic receptors.
This is evident both in an increase in the response of DA- (and Ne-)
sensitive adenylate cyclase to catecholaminergic agonists (Kalisker
et al., 1973; Mishra et al., 1974), and an increase in the number of
apparent receptors (Creese, Burt, & Snyder, 1977; Sporn, Wolfe,
Harden, & Molinoff, 1977). These changes presumably underlie the
gradual increase over time that occurs in the amount of motor activity elicited by apomorphine in 6-HDA-treated rats with DA depletions
in excess of 80 percent. This can be seen in Figure 3. As with
the loss of high-affinity DA-uptake sites, this increase in target
cell sensitivity should enhance the efficacy of released transmitter
and thereby lessen the functional impact of the brain lesions.

To summarize, DA-depleting brain lesions appear to provoke several adaptive changes which reduce the functional impact of the lesions. Some of them occur soon after the lesion, others take place
slowly, but collectively they serve to maintain dopaminergic neurotransmission despite the loss of a substantial portion of the nerve
terminals. Indeed, the apparent absence of an increase in target cell
sensitivity in animals with DA-depletions of up to 80 percent may sig-
nify that the postsynaptic cells continue to receive adequate dopaminergic input even after a lesion of this magnitude. This is presumably

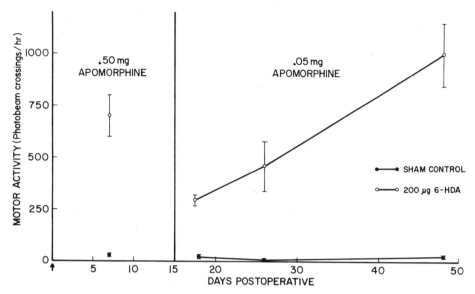

Fig. 3.   Apomorphine-induced motor activity in 6-HDA-treated rats
with large DA-depletions (87-95%), as a function of days
since treatment (arrow). Apomorphine was administered ip
5 min prior to testing. Motor activity was measured as
the number of photobeam crossings during the first hour
of testing. By the seventh postoperative day, the response
to apomorphine (.5 mg/kg) was significantly elevated in the
lesioned animals (o), but not in the controls (●). Thereafter, the response to apomorphine (.05 mg/kg) continued to
increase for at least 48 days postoperatively. Each point
represents the mean ± S.E.M. for 4-7 rats (Zigmond &
Stricker, 1980)

facilitated by the increase in DA turnover in residual terminals and
by an increase in diffusion of DA resulting from the loss of reuptake
sites. Although these processes may not maintain DA receptor activation at normal levels when DA-depletions exceed 80 percent, it is not
until DA-depletions are 90-95 percent or greater that animals become
akinetic, cataleptic, and show marked sensory neglect for prolonged
periods of time. Thus, the rapid compensatory neurochemical changes
that occur after the lesions are evidently so effective that the disruption in dopaminergic neurotransmission must be near-total before
gross behavioral dysfunctions are observed. Yet, even then there can
be a gradual recovery of function due to more slowly developing neurochemical processes; that is, the progressive development of increased responsiveness of the postsynaptic cells to DA, and a possible increase in the capacity of the residual neurons to synthesize
and release DA. On the other hand, the inability of lesioned animals
to behave appropriately when stressed indicates that these adaptive

neurochemical changes, including the presence of postsynaptic supersensitivity, do not insure the return of completely normal function,
perhaps because the residual neurons are unable to provide sufficient
DA in response to increased need due to their already elevated rate
of DA turnover.

Implications

     Our discussion thus far has been based on empirical evidence
that indicates a special role for brain catecholamines in the mediation of motivated behavior. This role could also be derived from
consideration of the anatomical organization of these neurons and
the biochemical bases for regulation of their synaptic activities.
The distribution of the noradrenergic neurons in the brain clearly
resembles that of the sympathetic nervous system, in that both pathways have extensive branches which project to an exceptionally large
number of diverse structures from only a few cell groups. This arrangement, whereby long axons and collaterals originating in the
locus coeruleus can spread nervous activity simultaneously to prac-
tically all portions of the cerebral and cerebellar cortices (Moore
& Bloom, 1979), is consistent with the postulated function of the
central noradrenergic fibers in mediating tonic electrocortical arousal and alertness (Jones, Bobillier, Pin, & Jouvet, 1973). Similarly, the DA-containing neurons arising from the substantia nigra send
their axons rostralward to many telencephalic structures, including
the corpus striatum, thus providing an anatomical basis for their influence on phasic extrapyramidal motor activities (Carlsson, 1959;
Jones et al., 1973). The precise neurophysiological nature of that
influence remains unclear. Some studies suggest that catecholamine-
containing neurons exert long-lasting inhibitory postsynaptic effects
(Connor, 1970; Hoffer, Siggins, Oliver, & Bloom, 1973). If so, then
impulses in these pathways may permit arousal by depressing activity
in structures normally exerting an inhibitory influence. More recently, it has been proposed that catecholamines often serve a per-
missive role, increasing the responsiveness of target cells to other
inputs (Moises, Woodward, Hoffer, & Freedman, 1979; Waterhouse &
Woodward, 1980). This suggests that activity in catecholaminergic
projections may promote arousal by facilitating the transmission of
sensory and/or motor signals.

     An important characteristic of these neurons is that they nor-
mally operate at a low and relatively constant frequency. As mentioned previously, the modulation of synaptic transmission by changes
in release and in target cell sensitivity tends to maintain activity
of catecholamine-containing pathways within a desired range under
basal conditions and to dampen the synaptic response to abrupt
changes in input. Furthermore, the catecholamines released into the
synapse do not directly affect ion channels, in contrast to the familiar effects of acetylcholine at the mammalian neuromuscular junc-

tion (i.e., it produces a rapid alteration of membrane conductance, generating a postjunctional potential of millisecond duration). Instead, they act through several intervening steps resulting in a much slower and more prolonged response. These characteristics would not be suited for the transmission of primary sensory information or messages in a final somatic motor pathway, in which rapid, high-fidelity transmission is necessary. However, they do seem appropriate to neural pathways subserving homeostasis and motivation, since transient changes in input must be ignored while sustained changes must evoke a gradual, coordinated response.

Catecholaminergic neurons normally synthesize transmitter at a rate well below their maximal potential, as defined by the availability of tyrosine hydroxylase (Lovenberg & Bruckwick, 1975). This permits intact animals to increase turnover rapidly in response to stimuli that increase the demand for catecholaminergic neurotransmission. To the extent that lesioned animals already have utilized a significant portion of this reserve capacity to elevate basal turnover in residual neurons, they will have compromised their ability to respond to increased demand. This may account for our observations that rats with very large DA-depleting brain lesions apparently do not increase DA release after haloperidol treatment by as much as control animals do, as illustrated in Table 2. Moreover, such brain-damaged

Table 2. Effect of Haloperidol on Striatal DOPAC Concentration in Control and 6-HDA Lesioned Rats[a,b]

Group (n)	Dopamine	DOPAC	$\dfrac{DOPAC}{DA}$
	(ug/gm)		
Control			
Saline (21)	11.88 ±.27	1.12 ±.36	.094 ±.002
Haloperidol (22)	10.79 ±.27	4.15 ±.16	.387 ±.015
Lesioned			
Saline (10)	.58 ±.07	.14 ±.02	.251 ±.034
Haloperidol (11)	.66 ±.08	.28 ±.03	.441 ±.024

[a] Lesioned rats received DMI (25 mg/kg, i.p.) and two injections of 6-HDA (250 ug, ivt.) 30 and 45 min. later.

[b] Animals received 1 mg/kg (s.c.) haloperidol and were sacrificed 1 hr. later.

All values represent the means ± S.E.M.

rats do not build nests or increase food intake when exposed to intense cold, or increase water and salt consumption following the loss
of plasma volume, but instead regress to an akinetic and cataleptic
state as they do when a dopaminergic antagonist is given (Stricker
et al., 1975; Stricker, 1976; Van Zoeren & Stricker, 1977).

To summarize, we have proposed that the anatomical and biochemical characteristics of catecholaminergic systems make unique and non-
transferable their function in mediating the activational component
of homeostatic responses. They also provide explanations for the surprising absence of major functional deficits despite extensive damage
to the systems, for the recovery of function that can occur even when
the damage is almost complete, and for their relative insensitivity
to weak stimuli as well as their residual intolerance of intense
stimuli. Inasmuch as this analysis appears to account for many aspects of the behavior of our brain-damaged animals, we are encouraged
to believe it may also shed some light on the etiology, detection, and
treatment of certain related dysfunctions in human patients.

Parkinsons's Disease. The best documented example of a human
dysfunction involving the loss of central catecholaminergic neurons
is Parkinsonism, a neurological disease affecting approximately 1
percent of the population over 50 years of age. Upon autopsy, Parkinsonian patients invariably have a marked loss of DA-containing
cells in the substantia nigra, a more moderate loss of NE-containing
cells in the locus coeruleus, and extensive catecholamine depletions
in several brain regions, particularly the basal ganglia (Bernheimer,
Birkmayer, Hornykiewicz, Jellinger, & Seitelberger, 1973). As indicated above, large DA-depleting brain lesions in rats lead to a syndrome including most of the cardinal extrapyramidal symptoms of Parkinsonism; namely, akinesia, muscular rigidity, and postural disorders (i.e., all but tremor). In addition, we have found that lesioned
rats show no prominent symptoms until DA-depletions exceed 90-95 percent, that "paradoxical kinesia" results when the animals are exposed
to various brief activating situations, and that increased symptoms
occur when the rats are confronted with physiological or psychological stress. Each of these characteristics parallel phenomena that
are well documented in patients with Parkinson's disease. Thus, mild
cases of Parkinsonism are accompanied by 70-80 percent decreases in
striatal DA, whereas severe symptomatology is associated with DA-depletions of 90 percent or greater (Bernheimer et al., 1973). Moreover, a brief period of marked improvement sometimes occurs when Parkinsonian patients are presented with certain emergencies. For example, patients who have been akinetic for years have been reported
to run from a burning building, and to return to their previous unresponsive condition when they reach safety moments later. Stress
commonly exacerbates otherwise mild symptoms, as in the case of patients whose motor performance worsens when they become angry (Schwab
& Zieper, 1965).

We believe that the lack of neurological deficits, despite sig-nificant neuronal damage, can be explained in terms of the compensa-tory changes which occur in residual neurons (Hornykiewicz, 1979), and that these changes have implications for the seemingly contra-dictory effects of stress as well. For a brief period an intense stimulus might be expected to increase transmitter release suffici-ently to restore function. However, if DA release exceeds the capac-ity for synthesis, stores eventually will be depleted and function should be once again impaired. These hypotheses are, of course, de-rived from our work with brain-damaged rats, although there is an ob-vious point of contrast between the abrupt loss of dopaminergic nerve terminals in those animals and the gradually increasing neuropathy that is presumed to occur in patients with Parkinson's Disease. Nev-ertheless, an insidious loss of functional neurons that progressed over the years would provide ample time for the compensatory changes outlined above to develop. Indeed, significant increases in the ratios of homovanillic acid (another DA metabolite) to DA and tyro-sine hydroxylase activity to DA, and in apparent DA receptor number, all have been observed to parallel decreases in striatal DA in autopsy material obtained from patients who died with advanced Parkinsonism (Bernheimer et al., 1973; Lloyd, Davidson, & Hornykiewicz, 1975; Lee, Seeman, Rajput, Farley, & Hornykiewicz, 1978).

This perspective has clear implications for the detection of Parkinson's Disease in individuals with, as yet, few neurological symptoms. The performance of those subjects on various tasks should be unusually susceptible to disruption, such as by increasing task complexity or distracting stimulation, especially when damage to dopa-minergic neurons is relatively large. Similarly, the behavioral re-sponses of such subjects should be more severely affected following treatment with drugs that decrease dopaminergic activity (such as α-methyltyrosine or spiroperidol), while unusual increase in be-havioral arousal might be expected following treatment with drugs that increase dopaminergic activity (such as L-dopa or apomorphine).

This perspective also provides a rationale for the effective use of L-dopa in the symptomatic treatment of Parkinsonism by correcting the striatal DA deficiency. Unlike DA, L-dopa (the amino acid precur-sor in the biosynthesis of DA) can cross the blood-brain barrier. Ap-parently it is largely converted to DA in striatal microvessels (Mela-med, Hefti, & Wurtman, 1980a) and interneurons or efferents (Duvoisin, & Mytilineou, 1978; Melamed et al., 1980b). Thus, the DA formed in the brain is not simply synthesized within residual terminals, aug-menting the relatively small amounts of DA that are synthesized and released from dopaminergic terminals. Instead, the DA is formed throughout the CNS, and thereby able to act in a hormonal fashion within the denervated area. Unfortunately, it is difficult to gauge the dose of L-dopa required to deliver an appropriate amount of DA to this target site, and if relatively large doses of L-dopa are taken they might be expected to reduce receptor sensitivity and/or DA re-

lease from residual dopaminergic neurons, and thereby limit the effectiveness of the treatment, perhaps contributing to the "on-off"
phenomenon (Lee et al., 1978). For the same reason, during periodic
lapses in L-dopa treatment, Parkinsonian patients may be left temporarily in considerably worse shape than they would have been in the absence of any treatment. Since DA synthesis is limited by the rate of
tyrosine hydroxylation and can be increased by providing additional
amounts of the substrates for this reaction, including tyrosine and
pterin cofactor, the treatment of mild Parkinsonism by the systemic
administration of these substances might provide an advantage over
L-dopa treatment because additional DA would be formed only within
residual DA terminals. In this way, the availability of TH enzyme
would restrict the rate of formation, and thus release, of DA. This
arrangement would be consistent with our model in which DA formed
from residual dopaminergic terminals in brain-damaged rats diffuses
to distant target cells and, in doing so, promotes recovery of function.

   Minimal Brain Dysfunction. Minimal Brain Dysfunction is a behavioral syndrome diagnosed in up to 5 to 10 percent of school-age
children. Its characteristic features include hyperactivity, dis-
tractability, and short attention span, as well as certain perceptual-
cognitive signs. The neural correlates of this condition are unknown,
as such children typically fail to show classical signs of organic
brain damage and even soft neurological signs may be absent. However,
it is noteworthy that the World War I pandemic of influenza sometimes
produced a postencephalitic Parkinsonian syndrome in adults and a behavioral syndrome in children resembling Minimal Brain Dsyfunction
(Hohman, 1922). These observations imply that a deficiency in central
catecholaminergic function may also be common to both syndromes. Consistent with this hypothesis are the findings that the levels of homovanillic acid in the cerebrospinal fluid of children with Minimal
Brain Dysfunction are significantly lower than those found in control
subjects (Shaywitz, Cohen, & Bowers, 1977). Furthermore, this disorder often is associated with perinatal hypoxia, a condition found
to damage central catecholaminergic neurons (Zervas, Hori, Negora,
Wurtman, Larin, & Lavyne, 1974; Wender, 1975; Robinson, & Coyle,
1980). It is important to note, in this regard, that such damage
would fail to be detected by conventional histological analyses,
even upon autopsy, because the axons and terminals of aminergic neurons are both too thin and too diffuse (Wolf, Stricker, & Zigmond,
1978).

   Like Parkinsonian patients, children with Minimal Brain Dsyfunction are similar in certain ways to the animal model we have described. For example, while the behavioral difficulties seen in Minimal
Brain Dysfunction tend to lessen with age, they persist into adolescence and adult life (Wood, Reimherr, Wender, & Johnson, 1976). Furthermore, they often can be ameliorated by continual use of pharmacological stimulants, especially catecholaminergic agonists such as

amphetamine, methylphenidate, and caffeine (Bradley, 1950; Millichap, 1973). Moreover, such children are unusually sensitive to the disruptive effects of stressful environments, and fatigue easily (Wender, 1975; Zentall, 1975).

Assuming that some early and persistent cerebral DA deficiency is associated with Minimal Brain Dysfunction, a more appropriate animal model might involve neonatal DA-depletion. It is, therefore, of interest that in the normal course of development, prepubertal hyperkinesis in rats is observed in association with the incomplete dopaminergic innervation of the forebrain. Moreover, intracisternal or intraventricular treatment of neonatal rat pups with 6-HDA prevents the attainment of adult levels of brain catecholamines and prolongs that period of hyperkinesis (Shaywitz, Yager, & Klopper, 1976; Erinoff, MacPhail, Heller, & Seiden, 1979), whereas treatment with amphetamine or methylphenidate reduces the increase of motor activity (Shaywitz, Klopper, Yager, & Gordon, 1976; Shaywitz, Klopper, & Gordon, 1978). It is interesting to note that the DA depletions were less than 60 percent in these animals, which might be expected from the effectiveness of indirect dopaminergic agonists like amphetamine and methylphenidate. These results are suggestive, although it remains to be determined whether the moderate DA-depleting brain lesions in rats also produces dysfunctions reminiscent of the cognitive features of Minimal Brain Dysfunction.

While the hyperkinetic symptoms associated with Minimal Brain Dysfunction have been interpreted as a sign of overarousal, the parallels with animals sustaining DA-depleting lesions, and particularly the efficacy of pharmacological stimulation, suggest the converse. In fact, phenobarbital in doses sedative to most control children are known to exacerbate the hyperactivity of children with Minimal Brain Dysfunction (Bradley, 1950; Wender, 1971). Moreover, electrophysiological and psychophysiological signs of underarousal have been reported in the latter group (Wikler, Dixon, & Parker, 1970; Satterfield, & Dawson, 1971). Thus, hyperactivity may represent a behavioral compensation which serves to heighten arousal levels and which becomes unnecessary under proper environmental conditions or following stimulant drug medication.

Summary and Conclusions

Observations from this and other laboratories indicate that damage to catecholamine-containing projections is not associated with gross behavioral impairments in rats until the loss of amine is considerable. This appears due, in part, to compensatory adjustments at residual catecholaminergic synapses and in other, interrelated pathways. However, while these adaptive changes permit apparently normal behavior under neutral laboratory conditions, the range of stimuli to which the animals will respond is reduced. Such animals are relatively unresponsive to mild stimuli and intolerant of intense ones. This may result from the small number of residual catecholamine-containing terminals, and the inability of those terminals to increase significantly their rate of transmitter release, respectively.

Animals with catecholamine-depleting brain lesions have several features which are reminiscent of human patients with Parkinson's Disease or Minimal Brain Dysfunction. These include a lack of correspondence between presumed central damage and neurological deficits, a temporary improvement in performance with increased stimulus intensity or catecholaminergic agonists, and an increased susceptibility to the disruptive effects of stress. The latter characteristic can be used to detect the dysfunctions in human subjects with subclinical brain damage and to assess the severity of the problem. Conversely, because the neurochemical adaptations contract the range of stimuli which elicit an optimal performance, in therapy the human subject should be alerted to the subtle differences in task complexity, emotional upset, and environmental stimulation that will promote or hinder his behavioral capabilities.

REFERENCES

Acheson, A.L., & Zigmond, M.J. Short and long-term changes in tyrosine hydroxylase activity in rat brain after subtotal destruction of central noradrenergic neurons. Journal of Neuroscience, 1981, 1, 493-504.
Acheson, A.L., Zigmond, M.J., & Stricker, E.M. Tyrosine hydroxylase and DOPAC in striatum after 6-hydroxydopamine. Transactions of the American Society for Neurochemistry, 1979, 10, 142.
Acheson, A.L., Zigmond, M.J., & Stricker, E.M. Compensatory increase in tyrosine hydroxylase activity in rat brain after intraventricular injections of 6-hydroxydopamine. Science, 1980, 207, 537-540.
Agid, Y., Javoy, F., & Glowinski, J. Hyperactivity of remaining dopaminergic neurons after partial destruction of the nigro-striatal dopaminergic system in the rat. Nature New Biology, 1973, 245, 150-151.
Anand, B.K., & Brobeck, J.R. Localization of a "feeding center" in the hypothalamus of the rat. Proceedings of the Society for Experimental Biology and Medicine, 1951, 77, 323-324.
Anden, N.E., Dahlstrom, A., Fuxe, K., Larsson, K., Olson, L., & Ungerstedt, U. Ascending monoamine neurons to the teleencephalon and diencephalon. Acta Physiologica Scandinavica, 1966, 67, 313-326.
Antelman, S.M., Rowland, N.E., & Fisher, A.E. Stress related recovery from lateral hypothalamic aphagia. Brain Research, 1976, 102, 346-350.
Bernheimer, H., Birkmayer, W., Hornykiewicz, O., Jellinger, K., & Seitelberger, F. Brain dopamine and the syndromes of Parkinson

and Huntington: Clinical, morphological and neurochemical correlations. Journal of the Neurological Sciences, 1973, 20, 415-
455.

Bjorklund, A., Baumgarten, H.G., & Rensch, A.   5,7-dihydroxytrypta-
mine: Improvement of its selectivity for serotonin neurons in
the CNS by pretreatment with desipramine. Journal of Neurochemistry, 1975, 24, 833-835.

Bradley, C.   Benzedrine and dexedrine in the treatment of children's
behaviour disorders.   Pediatrics, 1950, 5, 24-37.

Caggiula, A.R., Shaw, D.H., Antelman, S.M., & Edwards, D.J.   Interactive effects of brain catecholamines and variations in sexual
and non-sexual arousal on copulatory behavior of male rats.
Brain Research, 1976, 111, 321-336.

Carlsson, A.   The occurrence, distribution and physiological role of
catecholamines in the nervous system.   Pharmacological Reviews,
1959, 11, 490-493.

Cannon, W.B., & Rosenblueth, A.   The supersensitivity of denervated
structures.   New York: Macmillan, 1949.

Chiodo, L.A., Antelman, S.M., Caggiula, A.R., & Lineberry, C.G.   Sensory stimuli alter the discharge rate of dopamine (DA) neurons:
Evidence for two functional types of DA cells in the substantia
nigra.   Brain Research, 1980, 189, 544-549.

Connor, J.D.   Caudate nucleus neurons: Correlation of the effects of
substantia nigra stimulation with iontophoretic dopamine.   Journal of Physiology, 1970, 208, 691-703.

Cooper, B.R., Breese, G.R., Howard, J.L., & Grant, L.D.   Effect of
central catecholamine alterations by 6-hydroxydopamine on shuttle
box avoidance acquisition.   Physiology and Behavior, 1972, 9,
727-731.

Creese, I., Burt, D.R., & Snyder, S.H.   Dopamine receptor binding enhancement accompanies lesion-induced behavioral supersensitivity.
Science, 1977, 197, 596-598.

Duvoisin, R.C., & Mytilineou, C.   Where is L-DOPA decarboxylated in
the striatum after 6-hydroxydopamine nigrotomy?   Brain Research,
1978, 152, 369-373.

Epstein, A.N., & Teitelbaum, P.   Specific loss of the hypoglycemic
control of feeding in recovered lateral rats.   American Journal
of Physiology, 1967, 213, 1159-1167.

Erinoff, L., MacPhail, R.C., Heller, A., & Seiden, L.S.   Age-depen-
dent effects of 6-hydroxydopamine on locomotor activity in the
rat.   Brain Research, 1979, 164, 195-205.

Fibiger, H.C., Zis, A.P., & McGeer, E.G.   Feeding and drinking deficits after 6-hydroxydopamine administration in the rat: Similarities to the lateral hypothalamic syndrome.   Brain Research,
1973, 55, 135-148.

Hedreen, J.C., & Chalmers, J.P.   Neuronal degeneration in rat brain
induced by 6-hydroxydopamine: A histological and biochemical
study.   Brain Research, 1972, 47, 1-36.

Heffner, T.G., Zigmond, M.J., & Stricker, E.M.   Effects of dopaminergic agonists and antagonists on feeding in intact and 6-

hydroxydopamine-treated rats. Journal of Pharmacology and Experimental Therapeutics, 1977, 201, 386-399.

Hefti, F., Melamed, E., & Wurtman, R.J. Partial lesions of the dopaminergic nigrostriatal system in rat brain: Biochemical characterization. Brain Research, 1980, 195, 123-137.

Hoffer, B.J., Siggins, G.R., Oliver, A.P., & Bloom, F.E. Activation of the pathway from locus coeruleus to rat cerebellar Purkinje neurons: Pharmacological evidence of noradrenergic central inhibition. Journal of Pharmacology and Experimental Therapeutics, 1973, 184, 553-569.

Hohman, L.B. Post-encephalitic behavior disorders in children. Johns Hopkins Hospital Bulletin, 1922, 380, 373-375.

Hornykiewicz, O. Compensatory biochemical changes at the striatal dopamine synapse in Parkinson's disease--Limitations of L-DOPA therapy. In L.J. Poirier, T.L. Sourkes, & P.J. Bedard (Eds.), Advances in neurology. New York: Raven, 1979.

Jones, B.E., Bobillier, P., Pin, C., & Jouvet, M. The effect of lesions of catecholamine-containing neurons upon monoamine content of the brain and EEG and behavioral waking in the cat. Brain Research, 1973, 58, 157-177.

Kalisker, A., Rutledge, C.O., & Perkins, J.P. Effect of nerve degeneration by 6-hydroxydopamine on catecholamine-stimulated adenosine 3', 5'-monophosphate formation in rat cerebral cortex. Molecular Pharmacology, 1973, 9, 619-629.

Lee, T., Seeman, P., Rajput, A., Farley, I.J., & Hornykiewicz, O. Receptor basis for dopaminergic supersensitivity in Parkinson's disease. Nature, 1978, 273, 59-61.

Levitt, D.R., & Teitelbaum, P. Somnolence, akinesia, and sensory activation of motivated behavior in the lateral hypothalamic syndrome. Proceedings of the National Academy of Sciences, 1975, 72, 2819-2823.

Ljungberg, T., & Ungerstedt, U. Reinstatement of eating by dopamine agonists in aphagic dopamine denervated rats. Physiology and Behavior, 1976, 16, 277-283.

Lloyd, K.G., Davidson, L., & Hornykiewicz, O. The neurochemistry of Parkinsons' disease: Effect of L-DOPA therapy. Journal of Pharmacology and Experimental Therapeutics, 1975, 195, 453-464.

Lovenberg, W., & Bruckwick, E.A. Mechanisms of receptor mediated regulation of catecholamine synthesis in brain. In W.E. Bunney, Jr., & E. Usdin (Eds.), Pre- and postsynaptic receptors. New York: Marcel Dekker, 1975.

Marshall, J.F. Somatosensory inattention after dopamine-depleting intracerebral 6-OHDA injections: Spontaneous recovery and pharmacological control. Brain Research, 1979, 177, 311-324.

Marshall, J.F., Levitan, D., & Stricker, E.M. Activation-induced restoration of sensorimotor functions in rats with dopamine-depleting brain lesions. Journal of Comparative and Physiological Psychology, 1976, 90, 536-546.

Marshall, J.F., & Teitelbaum, P. Further analysis of sensory inattention following lateral hypothalamic damage in rats. Journal of Comparative and Physiological Psychology, 1974, 86, 375-395.

McGeer, E.G., & McGeer, P.L. Duplication of biochemical changes of Huntington's chorea by intrastriatal injections of glutamic and kainic acids. Nature, 1976, 263, 517-519.

Melamed, E., Hefti, F., & Wurtman, R.J. Decarboxylation of exogenous L-DOPA in rat striatum after lesions of the dopaminergic nigro-striatal neurons: The role of striatal capillaries. Brain Research, 1980a, 198, 244-248.

Melamed, E., Hefti, F., & Wurtman, R.J. Diminished decarboxylation of L-DOPA in rat striatum after intrastriatal injections of kainic acid. Neuropharmacology, 1980b, 19, 409-411.

Millichap, J.G. Drugs in management of minimal brain dysfunction. Annals of the New York Academy of Sciences, 1973, 205, 321-334.

Mishra, R.K., Gardner, E.L., Katzman, R., & Makman, M.H. Enhancement of dopamine-stimulated adenylate cyclase activity in rat caudate after lesions in substantia nigra: Evidence for denervation supersensitivity. Proceedings of the National Academy of Sciences, 1974, 71, 3883-3887.

Moises, H.C., Woodward, D.J., Hoffer, B.J., & Freedman, R. Interactions of norepinephrine with Purkinje cell responses to putative amino acid neurotransmitters applied by microiontophoresis. Experimental Neurology, 1979, 64, 493-515.

Moore, R.Y., Bhatnagar, R.K., & Heller, A. Anatomical and chemical studies of a nigro-neostriatal projection in the cat. Brain Research, 1971, 30, 119-135.

Moore, R.Y., & Bloom, F.E. Central catecholamine neuron systems: Anatomy and physiology of the norepinephrine and epinephrine systems. Annual Review of Neuroscience, 1979, 2, 113-168.

Nieoullon, A., Cheramy, A., & Glowinski, J. Nigral and striatal dopamine release under sensory stimuli. Nature, 1977, 269, 340-342.

Oltmans, G.A., & Harvey, J.A. LH syndrome and brain catecholamine levels after lesions of the nigrostriatal bundle. Physiology and Behavior, 1972, 8, 69-78.

Peterson, G.M., & Moore, R.Y. Selective effects of kainic acid on diencephalic neurons. Brain Research, 1980, 202, 165-182.

Powley, T.L., & Keesey, R.E. Relationship of body weight to the lateral hypothalamic feeding syndrome. Journal of Comparative and Physiological Psychology, 1970, 70, 25-36.

Reis, D.J., Joh, T.H., & Ross, R.A. Effects of reserpine on activities and amounts of tyrosine hydroxylase and dopamine-β-hydroxylase in catecholamine neuronal systems in rat brain. Journal of Pharmacology and Experimental Therapeutics, 1975, 193, 775-784.

Robinson, R.G., & Coyle, J.T. The differential effect of right versus left hemispheric cerebral infarction on catecholamines and behavior in the rat. Brain Research, 1980, 188, 63-78.

Saller, C.F., & Stricker, E.M. Gastrointestinal motility and body weight gain in rats after brain serotonin depletion by 5,7-dihydroxytryptamine. Neuropharmacology, 1978, 17, 499-506.

Satterfield, J.H., & Dawson, M.E. Electrodermal correlates of hyper-
    activity in children. Psychophysiology, 1971, 8, 191-197.
Schwab, R.S., & Zieper, I. Effects of mood, motivation, stress and
    alertness on the performance in Parkinson's disease. Psychia-
    tria et Neurologia, 1965, 150, 345-357.
Schwarcz, R., & Coyle, J.T. Striatal lesions with kainic acid: Neu-
    rochemical characteristics. Brain Research, 1977, 127, 235-249.
Seeman, P. Brain dopamine receptors. Pharmacological Reviews, 1980,
    32, 229-313.
Shaywitz, B.A., Cohen, D.J., & Bowers, M.B.,Jr. CSF monoamine metab-
    olites in children with minimal brain dysfunction: Evidence for
    alteration of brain dopamine. Journal of Pediatrics, 1977, 90,
    67-71.
Shaywitz, B.A., Klopper, J.H., & Gordon, J.W. Methylphenidate in
    6-hydroxydopamine-treated developing rat pups. Archives of
    Neurology, 1978, 35, 463-469.
Shaywitz, B.A., Klopper, J.H., Yager, R.D., & Gordon, J.W. Paradox-
    ical response to amphetamine in developing rats treated with
    6-hydroxydopamine. Nature, 1976, 261, 153-155.
Shaywitz, B.A., Yager, R.D., & Klopper, J.H. Selective brain dopa-
    mine depletion in developing rats: An experimental model of
    minimal brain dysfunction. Science, 1976, 191, 305-308.
Snyder, A.M., Stricker, E.M., & Zigmond, M.J. Stress-induced neuro-
    logical impairments after 6-hydroxydopamine: Effect of lesion
    size and age. Society for Neuroscience Abstracts, 1980, 6, 91.
Sporn, J.R., Wolfe, B.B., Harden, T.K., & Molinoff, P.B. Supersen-
    sitivity in rat cerebral cortex: Pre- and post-synaptic effects
    of 6-hydroxydopamine at noradrenergic synapses. Molecular
    Pharmacology, 1977, 13, 1170-1180.
Stricker, E.M. Drinking by rats after lateral hypothalamic lesions:
    A new look at the lateral hypothalamic syndrome. Journal of
    Comparative and Physiological Psychology, 1976, 90, 127-143.
Stricker, E.M., Cooper, P.H., Marshall, J.F., & Zigmond, M.J. Acute
    homeostatic imbalances reinstate sensorimotor dysfunctions in
    rats with lateral hypothalamic lesions. Journal of Comparative
    and Physiological Psychology, 1979, 93, 512-521.
Stricker, E.M., Friedman, M.I., & Zigmond, M.J. Glucoregulatory
    feeding by rats after intraventricular 6-hydroxydopamine or
    lateral hypothalamic lesions. Science, 1975, 189, 895-897.
Stricker, E.M., Swerdloff, A.F., & Zigmond, M.J. Intrahypothalamic
    injections of kainic acid produce feeding and drinking deficits
    in rats. Brain Research, 1978, 158, 470-473.
Stricker, E.M., & Wolf, G. The effects of hypovolemia on drinking
    in rats with lateral hypothalamic damage. Proceedings of the
    Society for Experimental Biology and Medicine, 1967, 124, 816-
    820.
Stricker, E.M., & Zigmond, M.J. Effects on homeostasis of intraven-
    tricular injection of 6-hydroxydopamine in rats. Journal of
    Comparative and Physiological Psychology, 1974, 86, 973-994.
Stricker, E.M., & Zigmond, M.J. Recovery of function following

damage to central catecholamine-containing neurons: A neurochemical model for the lateral hypothalamic syndrome. In J.
M. Sprague & A.N. Epstein (Eds.), Progress in psychobiology
and physiological psychology. New York: Academic Press, 1976.

Teitelbaum, P., & Epstein, A.N. The lateral hypothalamic syndrome:
Recovery of feeding and drinking after lateral hypothalamic
lesions. Psychological Reviews, 1962, 69, 74-90.

Ungerstedt, U. Adipsia and aphagia after 6-hydroxydopamine induced
degeneration of the nigro-striatal dopamine system. Acta Physiologica Scandinavica, 1971, Suppl. 367, 95-122.

Uretsky, N.J., & Iversen, L.L. Effects of 6-hydroxydopamine on catecholamine containing neurones in the rat brain. Journal of
Neurochemistry, 1970, 17, 269-278.

Van Zoeren, J.G., & Stricker, E.M. Effects of preoptic, lateral
hypothalamic, or dopamine-depleting lesions on behavioral ther-
moregulation in rats exposed to the cold. Journal of Comparative and Physiological Psychology, 1977, 91, 989-999.

Waterhouse, B.D., & Woodward, D.J. Interaction of norepinephrine
with cerebrocortical activity evoked by stimulation of somatosensory afferent pathways in the rat. Experimental Neurology,
1980, 67, 11-34.

Wender, P.H. Minimal brain dysfunction in children. New York:
Wiley & Sons, 1971.

Wender, P.H. The minimal brain dysfunction syndrome. Annual Review
of Medicine, 1975, 26, 45-62.

Westerink, B.H.C. The effects of drugs on dopamine biosynthesis and
metabolism in the brain. In A.S. Horn, J. Korf, & B.H.C. Westerink (Eds.), The neurobiology of dopamine. New York: Academic
Press, 1979.

Wikler, A., Dixon, J.F., & Parker, J.B. Brain function in problem
children and controls: Psychometric, neurological, and electroencephalographic comparison. American Journal of Psychiatry,
1970, 127, 634-645.

Wolf, G., Stricker, E.M., & Zigmond, M.J. Brain lesions: Induction,
analysis and the problem of recovery of function. In S. Finger
(Ed.), Recovery from brain damage. New York: Plenum, 1978.

Wood, D.R., Reimherr, F.W., Wender, P.H., & Johnson, G.E. Diagnosis
and treatment of minimal brain dysfunction in adults. Archives
of General Psychiatry, 1976, 33, 1453-1460.

Zentall, S. Optimal stimulation as theoretical basis of hyperactivity. American Journal of Orthopsychiatry, 1975, 45, 549-463.

Zervas, N.T., Hori, H., Negora, M., Wurtman, R.J., Larin, F., &
Lavyne, M.H. Reduction in brain dopamine following experimental
ischaemia. Nature, 1974, 247, 283-284.

Zigmond, M.J., Heffner, T.G., & Stricker, E.M. The effect of altered
dopaminergic activity on food intake in the rat: Evidence for an
optimal level of dopaminergic activity for behavior. Progress
in Neuro-Psychopharmacology, 1980, 4, 351-362.

Zigmond, M.J., & Stricker, E.M. Deficits in feeding behavior after
intraventricular injection of 6-hydroxydopamine in rats. Science, 1972, 177, 1211-1214.

Zigmond, M.J., & Stricker, E.M. Recovery of feeding and drinking by
    rats after intraventricular 6-hydroxydopamine or lateral hypo-
    thalamic lesions. Science, 1973, 182, 717-720.
Zigmond, M.J., & Stricker, E.M. Ingestive behavior following damage
    to central dopamine neurons: Implications for homeostasis and
    recovery of function. In E. Usdin (Ed.), Neuropsychopharmacology
    of monoamines and their regulatory enzymes. New York: Raven,
    1974.
Zigmond, M.J., & Stricker, E.M. Supersensitivity after intraventricu-
    lar 6-hydroxydopamine: Relation to dopamine depletion. Experi-
    entia, 1980, 36, 436-437.
Zivkovic, B., Guidotti, A., & Costa, E. Effects of neuroleptics on
    striatal tyrosine hydroxylase: Changes in affinity for the pter-
    dine cofactor. Molecular Pharmacology, 1974, 10, 727-735.

CONTRIBUTORS

Marilyn S. Albert
    Massachusetts General Hospital, Boston

François Boller
    Department of Psychiatry
    University of Pittsburgh School of Medicine

Nelson Butters
    Veterans Administration Medical Center, Boston
    Boston University School of Medicine

Carol Dorr
    Yale New Haven Hospital, New Haven, CT

Gerald Goldstein
    Highland Drive Veterans Administration Medical Center
    Pittsburgh

Nancy Helm-Estabrooks
    Veterans Administration Medical Center, Boston

Audrey L. Holland
    Department of Psychiatry
    University of Pittsburgh School of Medicine

Youngjai Kim
    Department of Psychiatry
    University of Pittsburgh School of Medicine

Patti Miliotis
    Veterans Administration Medical Center, Boston
    Boston University School of Medicine

John Moossy
    Presbyterian University Hospital
    Pittsburgh

Oscar A. Parsons
    Department of Psychiatry and Behavioral Sciences
    University of Oklahoma Health Sciences Center

Eldred Richey
      University of Alabama Medical School, Mobile

Daniel S. Sax
      Boston University School of Medicine

Edward M. Stricker
      Departments of Biological Sciences, Psychology & Psychiatry
      University of Pittsburgh School of Medicine

Diane Wagener
      Department of Psychiatry
      University of Pittsburgh School of Medicine

Sidney K. Wolfson
      Montefiore Hospital
      Pittsburgh

Michael J. Zigmond
      Departments of Biological Sciences, Psychology & Psychiatry
      University of Pittsburgh School of Medicine

INDEX

Affective psychiatric disorders,
    71-74
Aging, *See* Alzheimer disease;
    Dementia; Elderly
Albumin, 95
Alcohol abuse, 19
Alcoholic Korsakoff's syndrome,
    See Alcoholism;
    Korsakoff's syndrome
Alcoholism, 4, 13-14, 98
  neuropsychology of, 77-81
  psychiatric disorders, 55-56
  sex differences, 35-36
Alzheimer disease, 4, 13, 89-114
  alcoholism and, 79
  assessment of, 97-106, 112-113
  cerebral blood flow and,
    109-110
  computed tomography and,
    109-111
  electroencephalography and,
    106-108
  epidemiology of, 89-91
  etiology and pathophysiology
    of, 91-96
  geropsychiatry, 75
  memory and, 144-145
  neurochemistry and, 111-112
  neuropathology, 112
  treatment, 76
  See also Dementia
Alzheimer-Fischer disease, 94
American Psychological Associa-
    tion, 20
Amnesia
  anterograde/retrograde memory
    deficits, 128-141

Amnesia (continued)
  memory deficits compared,
    141-142
  See also Memory
Anterograde memory deficits,
    128-141
Aphasia
  anterior/posterior special-
    ization, 9
  assessment and, 3-4
  dementia and, 100
  treatment of, 41-54
  See also Language
Apraxia, 101
Assessment and diagnosis
  affective disorders, 71-74
  alcoholism, 77-81
  Alzheimer disease, 89, 94-95,
    112-113
  basic principles of, 7-10
  dementia, 90, 91, 97-106,
    113-114
  dementia syndrome of depression,
    113-114
  future directions and, 14
  geropsychiatry, 74-77
  memory, 127-155
  multi-infarct dementia, 113
  neuropsychology and, 2-4, 6-7,
    21-26
  psychiatric disorders, 55-87
  schizophrenia, 58-65
  temporal lobe psychiatric
    disorders, 65-71
  See also Tests and testing
Asymmetries, 32-33
Attention (brain), 98

185